Management of Low Back Pain in Prim

Acquisitions editor: Geoff Smaldon
Development editor: Zoë A Youd
Production controller: Anthony Read
Desk editor: Jane Campbell
Cover designer: Fred Rose

Management of Low Back Pain in Primary Care

Edited by:

R. Bartley MSc MISCP MCSP
Chartered Physiotherapist, Duhallow Physiotherapy Clinic, Cork, Ireland

P. Coffey MRCP MRCGP
General Practitioner, Long Hanborough Surgery, Witney, Oxfordshire, UK

BUTTERWORTH
HEINEMANN

OXFORD   AUCKLAND   BOSTON   JOHANNESBURG   MELBOURNE   NEW DELHI

Butterworth-Heinemann
Linacre House, Jordan Hill, Oxford OX2 8DP
225 Wildwood Avenue, Woburn, MA 01801-2041
A division of Reed Educational and Professional Publishing Ltd

A member of the Reed Elsevier plc group

First published 2001

British Library Cataloguing in Publication Data
Management of low back pain in primary care
1. Backache
I. Bartley, R.   II. Coffey, P.
617.5'64'06

Library of Congress Cataloguing in Publication Data
Management of low back pain in primary care/edited by R. Bartley,
    P. Coffey.
    p. cm.
Includes bibliographical references and index.
ISBN 0 7506 4787 6
1. Backache.   2. Primary care (Medicine)
I. Bartley, R. (Richard)   II. Coffey, P. (Paul)
[DNLM: 1. Low Back Pain – therapy.   2. Low Back Pain –
diagnosis.   3. Primary Health Care – methods.
WE 755 M26635]
RD771.B217 M355
617.5'64–dc21   00–060887

ISBN 0 7506 4787 6

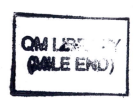

Composition by Genesis Typesetting, Laser Quay, Rochester, Kent
Printed and bound in Great Britain by MPG Books Ltd, Bodmin, Cornwall

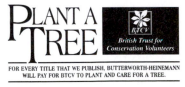

PLANT A TREE

British Trust for
Conservation Volunteers

FOR EVERY TITLE THAT WE PUBLISH, BUTTERWORTH-HEINEMANN
WILL PAY FOR BTCV TO PLANT AND CARE FOR A TREE.

Contents

List of Contibutors   vii
The RCGP clinical guidelines   ix
Introduction   xi

Section One   Background

1   GP Perspective and Management of Back Pain   3
    Paul Coffey

2   The Prevalence of Low Back Pain in Great Britain   19
    Paul Pynsent and Mark Webb

Section Two   Simple Back Pain

3   Simple Back Pain   29
    Richard Bartley

4   Rehabilitation of the Chronic Pain Patient   46
    Alison Hatfield and Richard Bartley

Section Three   Nerve Root Pain

5   Nerve Root Compression and Cauda Equina Syndrome   55
    Richard Bartley

6   Neurogenic Claudication and Spinal Stenosis   68
    Sunny Deo

Section Four   Suspected Serious Pathology

7   Inflammatory Causes of Low Back Pain   81
    Sally Edmonds

8   Neoplasms of the Spine   89
    Tom Cadoux-Hudson

9   Spinal Infection   99
    Andrew Wainwright

10   Metabolic Disorders of the Spine   106
Roger Smith

11   Management of Spinal Deformity in Primary Care   112
Jeremy Fairbank

Section Five   Investigations

12   Radiological Investigation and Management of Lumbosacral Pain   127
Paul O'Donnell and Eugene McNally

13   Laboratory Investigations for Low Back Pain   139
Daniel Porter

Section Six   Management

14   Drug Therapy in Acute and Chronic Low Back Pain in Primary Care   147
Andrew Cole

15   Spinal Surgery   153
James Wilson-MacDonald

16   Physical Therapy   163
Anthony Larcombe

17   The Role of the Specialist Physiotherapist   171
Patrick Hourigan

Epilogue

Implementation of the RCGP Clinical Guidelines   177
Christine A'Court

Glossary   189

Abbreviations   193

Index   195

Contributors

Christine A'Court MRCP MRCGP
General Practitioner
Carterton Surgery, Witney, Oxfordshire, UK

Richard Bartley MSc MISCP MCSP
Chartered Physiotherapist
Duhallow Physiotherapy Clinic, Cork, Ireland

Tom Cadoux-Hudson MB BS, D.Phil, FRCS, FRCS(SN)
Consultant Neurosurgeon
Radcliffe Infirmary, Oxford, UK

Paul Coffey MRCP, MRCGP
General Practitioner
Long Hanborough Surgery, Witney, Oxfordshire, UK

Andrew Cole BSc. MB BS FRCS (Tr and Orth)
Specialist Registrar in Trauma and Orthopaedics
Nuffield Orthopaedic Centre, Oxford, UK

Sunny Deo ChB FRCS (Tr and Orth)
Specialist Registrar in Trauma and Orthopaedics
Nuffield Orthopaedic Centre and John Radcliffe Hospital, Oxford, UK

Sally Edmonds MD FRCP
Consultant Rheumatologist
Nuffield Orthopaedic Centre, Oxford and Stoke Mandeville Hospital, Aylesbury, UK

Alison Hatfield MRCP
Consultant in Rehabilitation Medicine
Nuffield Orthopaedic Centre, Oxford, UK

Patrick Hourigan MMACP MCSP SRP
Chartered Physiotherapist
Princess Margaret Hospital, Exeter, UK

Jeremy CT Fairbank MD FRCS
Consultant Orthopaedic Surgeon
Nuffield Orthopaedic Centre, Oxford, UK

Anthony Larcombe DC BSc(Hons)
Chiropractor
Central Chiropractic Clinic, Oxford, UK

Eugene McNally MB (Hons) BCh BAO FRCR FRCPI
Consultant Radiologist
Nuffield Orthopaedic Centre, Oxford, UK

Paul G O'Donnell MRCP FRCR
Specialist Registrar in Radiology
Nuffield Orthopaedic Centre, Oxford, UK

Daniel Porter MB ChB, MD, BSc, FRCS(Ed), FRCS(Glasg)
Clinical Lecturer in Orthopaedic Surgery
Nuffield Department of Orthopaedic Surgery, University of Oxford,
Nuffield Orthopaedic Centre, Oxford, UK

Paul B. Pynsent PhD
Research Director
Research and Teaching Centre, Royal Orthopaedic Hospital,
Birmingham, UK

Roger Smith MA MD FRCP
Consultant Physician
Nuffield Orthopaedic Centre, Oxford, UK

Andrew M Wainwright BSc(Hons), MB, ChB, FRCS.
Specialist Registrar in Trauma and Orthopaedics
Nuffield Orthopaedic Centre, Oxford, UK

Mark R Webb FRCS
Specialist Registrar in Orthopaedics
Royal Orthopaedic Hospital, Birmingham, UK

James Wilson-MacDonald MCh FRCS
Consultant Orthopaedic Surgeon
Nuffield Orthopaedic Centre, Oxford, UK

The RCGP Clinical Guidelines for the Management of Acute Low Back Pain (February 1999)

A C U T E   L O W   B A C K   P A I N

DIAGNOSTIC TRIAGE

Diagnostic triage is the differential diagnosis between:

- Simple backache (non specific low back pain)
- Nerve root pain
- Possible serious spinal pathology

Simple backache: *specialist referral not required*

- Presentation 20-55 years
- Lumbosacral, buttocks & thighs
- "Mechanical" pain
- Patient well

Nerve root pain: *specialist referral not generally required within first 4 weeks, provided resolving*

- Unilateral leg pain worse than low back pain
- Radiates to foot or toes
- Numbness & paraesthesia in same distribution
- SLR reproduces leg pain
- Localised neurological signs

Red flags for possible serious spinal pathology: *consider prompt investigation or referral (less than 4 weeks)*

- Presentation under age 20 or onset over 55
- Non-mechanical pain
- Thoracic pain
- Past history - carcinoma, steroids, HIV
- Unwell, weight loss
- Widespread neurological symptoms or signs
- Structural deformity

Cauda equina syndrome: *emergency referral*

- Sphincter disturbance
- Gait disturbance
- Saddle anaesthesia

The evidence is weighed as follows:

*** Generally consistent finding in a majority of acceptable studies.

** Either based on a single acceptable study, or a weak or inconsistent finding in some of multiple acceptable studies.

* Limited scientific evidence, which does not meet all the criteria of 'acceptable' studies.

PRINCIPAL RECOMMENDATIONS

Assessment

- Carry out diagnostic triage (see left).
- X-rays are not routinely indicated in simple backache.
- Consider psychosocial 'yellow flags' (see over).

S I M P L E   B A C K A C H E

Drug Therapy

- Prescribe analgesics at regular intervals, not p.r.n.
- Start with paracetamol. If inadequate, substitute NSAIDs (eg ibuprofen or diclofenac) and then paracetamol-weak opioid compound (eg codydramol or coproxamol). Finally, consider adding a short course of muscle relaxant (eg diazepam or baclofen).
- Avoid strong opioids if possible.

Bed Rest

- Do not recommend or use bed rest as a treatment.
- Some patients may be confined to bed for a few days as a consequence of their pain but this should not be considered a treatment.

Advice on Staying Active

- Advise patients to stay as active as possible and to continue normal daily activities.
- Advise patients to increase their physical activities progressively over a few days or weeks.
- If a patient is working, then advice to stay at work or return to work as soon as possible is probably beneficial.

Manipulation

- Consider manipulative treatment for patients who need additional help with pain relief or who are failing to return to normal activities.

Back Exercises

- Referral for reactivation / rehabilitation should be considered for patients who have not returned to ordinary activities and work by 6 weeks.

EVIDENCE

* Diagnostic triage forms the basis for referral, investigation and management.
* Royal College of Radiologists Guidelines.
*** Psychosocial factors play an important role in low back pain and disability and influence the patient's response to treatment and rehabilitation.

** Paracetamol effectively reduces low back pain.
*** NSAIDs effectively reduce pain. Ibuprofen and diclofenac have lower risks of GI complications.
** Paracetamol-weak opioid compounds may be effective when NSAIDs or paracetamol alone are inadequate.
*** Muscle relaxants effectively reduce low back pain.

*** Bed rest for 2-7 days is worse than placebo or ordinary activity and is not as effective as alternative treatments for relief of pain, rate of recovery, return to daily activities and work.

*** Advice to continue ordinary activity can give equivalent or faster symptomatic recovery from the acute attack and lead to less chronic disability and less time off work.

*** Manipulation can provide short-term improvement in pain and activity levels and higher patient satisfaction.
** The optimum timing for this intervention is unclear.
** The risks of manipulation are very low in skilled hands.

*** It is doubtful that specific back exercises produce clinically significant improvement in acute low back pain.
** There is some evidence that exercise programmes and physical reconditioning can improve pain and functional levels in patients with chronic low back pain. There are theoretical arguments for starting this at around 6 weeks.

KEY PATIENT INFORMATION POINTS

◆ Simple Backache

– give positive messages

- There is nothing to worry about. Backache is very common.

- No sign of any serious damage or disease. Full recovery in days or weeks - but may vary.

- No permanent weakness. Recurrence possible - but does not mean re-injury.

- Activity is helpful, too much rest is not. Hurting does not mean harm.

◆ Nerve Root Pain

– give guarded positive messages

- No cause for alarm. No sign of disease.

- Conservative treatment should suffice - but may take a month or two.

- Full recovery expected - but recurrence possible.

◆ Possible Serious Spinal Pathology

– avoid negative messages

- Some tests are needed to make the diagnosis.

- Often these tests are negative.

- The specialist will advise on the best treatment.

- Rest or activity avoidance until appointment to see specialist.

PATIENT BOOKLET

The above messages can be enhanced by an educational booklet given at consultation. *The Back Book* is an evidence-based booklet developed for use with these guidelines, and is published by The Stationery Office (ISBN 011 702 0788).

These brief clinical guidelines and their supporting base of research evidence are intended to assist in the management of acute low back pain. It presents a synthesis of up-to-date international evidence and makes recommendations on case management.

Recommendations and evidence relate primarily to the first six weeks of an episode, when management decisions may be required in a changing clinical picture. However, the guidelines may also be useful in the sub-acute period.

These guidelines have been constructed by a multi-professional group and subjected to extensive professional review.

They are intended to be used as a guide by the whole range of health professionals who advise people with acute low back pain, particularly simple backache, in the NHS and in private practice.

Psychosocial 'Yellow Flags'

When conducting assessment, it may be useful to consider psychosocial 'yellow flags' (beliefs or behaviours on the part of the patient which may predict poor outcomes).

The following factors are important and consistently predict poor outcomes:

- a belief that back pain is harmful or potentially severely disabling

- fear-avoidance behaviour and reduced activity levels

- tendency to low mood and withdrawal from social interaction

- expectation of passive treatment(s) rather than a belief that active participation will help

Further information and copies of the full evidence base for these guidelines are available from:

Paula-Jayne McDowell,
Royal College of General Practitioners,
14 Princes Gate, Hyde Park, London, SW7 1PU
or at website - http://www.rcgp.org.uk

We are grateful to:
Professor Gordon Waddell
NHS Executive, Clinical Standards Advisory Group,
U.S. Agency for Health Care Policy & Research,
Swedish SBU, NZ National Health Committee

This document may be photocopied freely

GP62 2.99

With acknowledgements to the Royal College of General Practitioners.

Introduction

'Education is not that one knows more but that one behaves differently'

John Ruskin, 1819–1900

This book is written for general practitioners (GPs) and anyone involved in the initial management of patients with low back pain, particularly GP registrars, medical students, physiotherapists, chiropractors and osteopaths. Additionally it should provide a useful primary care perspective to providers of secondary care.

There are many times when a GP will feel slight dismay as it becomes clear why the patient has come for a consultation. This is either because the GP is not entirely confident about what is the best thing to do, or because there is little that can be done. Low back pain is one of the best examples of this because it is so common. One of the fundamental aims of this book is to enable the GP to feel both confident and positive (and ideally even enthusiastic) in his or her management of low back pain, which of course in practice is a very important part of the management of the patient per se.

The book is based on the experience of Richard Bartley who worked at the interface between primary and secondary care as a triage physiotherapist in the Back Pain Triage Clinic at the Nuffield Orthopaedic Centre in Oxford, and Paul Coffey who has been a 'front-line' GP for 20 years. Additionally, many chapters have been written by specialists and edited for primary care.

This book builds on the seminal RCGP guidelines on acute low back pain and examines the implications of primary care management. We do not advocate a mechanical adherence to the guidelines but rather suggest that they should be used as an educational tool to help manage individual patients better.

For the chiropractor, osteopath, and chartered physiotherapist, we hope this book will be a helpful review of current evidence-based practice, and that the more specialized chapters should give good insight into how secondary care is organized, so that when primary management fails to solve the problem he or she may be confident in explaining what will happen next to the patient. We hope that the book builds on the increasing recognition and understanding of each other's roles and skills in the care of patients with back problems in the community.

For many GPs, reading Chapters 1–6 may be sufficient to help in everyday management, dipping into the more specialized areas as needs arise and using the glossary as a reference. However, for the practitioner who is keenly interested in the subject, reading this book in its entirety should be a good investment. Each chapter is designed to be read on its own as time and interest permit. We make no apology therefore for the fact that many key issues appear in several chapters.

Note on terminology

Various nomenclature are used to describe the features of mechanical low back pain. These include 'simple back ache' and 'non-specific low back pain'.

Much erudite discussion took place in the pub between the authors as to which terminology should be used in this book. Like many other learned writers before, we could not come to an entirely satisfactory conclusion. None of the current terms accurately describe non-serious low back pain, in the way that can satisfy both clinician and patient.

Simple backache

This is emphasized in the 1996 RCGP clinical guidelines in an attempt to de-medicalize low back pain, and reassure sufferers and health care professionals that mechanical low back pain is rarely due to a serious cause. However critics of this approach argue that 'simple backache' could be misinterpreted as implying that all cases of low back pain are of minor inconvenience.

Whilst mechanical low back pain is usually self-limiting and long-term disability can be potentially avoided, lumbosacral pain can be severe and distressing. Recognising this distress, whilst providing appropriate reassurance and advice, may be more effective in preventing chronicity than simply dismissing the patient's suffering as being of little medical consequence. With an ever-increasing scepticism amongst the public towards the medical profession, empathy can go a long way in improving patient compliance.

Backache is also an unhelpful term. Patients frequently report pain rather than an ache to the GP. An acute episode of severe low back pain with the patient experiencing difficulty performing simple daily activities can hardly be described as an ache.

Non-specific low back pain

The term 'non-specific low back pain' avoids emotive words such as 'simple', and allows the clinician to avoid the need to label patients with plausible or spurious (and difficult to confirm) diagnoses, such as 'slipped discs' or 'joints out of place'. However it is meaningless to patients, being an example of medical jargon that conveys little to the patient about his or her condition.

This book draws on much of the RCGP clinical guidelines for the management of acute low back pain. The authors have therefore decided to keep close to the terminology used by the RCGP, i.e. simple backache for non-serious low back pain. However ache has been changed to pain.

Acknowledgements

We wish to thank all the contributors for helping us put this book together.

We are also grateful to Dr C A'Court MRCGP, Dr A Breen DC, Mr P Hourigan MCSP, Mr N Hunt DC, Dr E McNally FRCR, Dr Matthias Hickey FFR, RCSI, Dr S Stamp FRCGP and Professor G Waddell FRCS for their helpful advice, and in particular, Mr JCT Fairbank FRCS for his critical appraisal of a number of chapters.

Derek Bartley, Paul Cooper and Alison Davies provided excellent technical support and we wish to thank the following GPs for reviewing individual chapters; Dr D Bullock, Dr B Condon, Dr G Corrigan, Dr R Curtin, Dr J Devine, Dr J Keally, Dr T McCoy, Dr M Tangney.

Finally we wish to thank our wives, Jane and Maureen for their unstinting support.

RB and PC
April 2000

Background

Chapter 1

GP Perspective and Management of Back Pain

Paul Coffey

General practitioner perspective

Low back pain is now clearly established as a medical condition, with a few notable exceptions, and primary care management is starting to acknowledge that tenet.

Previous assumptions, for that was in effect all that many were, that the proper management depended on specialist surgical advice, be it orthopaedic or neurosurgical, are being dispelled. It is becoming realized that primary care management should assume a greater importance than hitherto, both in the care of acute presentations and in the prevention of chronic low back pain.

GPs and everyone else involved in looking after low back pain patients have always intuitively felt that the patient's attitudes and beliefs about healthcare and illness in general can have a huge affect on the outcome of treatment. It has been a great help to have this formally established and recently incorporated into the updated 1999 RCGP guidelines under the term psycho-social factors or 'Yellow Flags'.

Psychosocial 'Yellow Flags'

When conducting assessment, it may be useful to consider psychosocial 'yellow flags' (beliefs or behaviours on the part of the patient which may predict poor outcomes).

The following factors are important and consistently predict poor outcomes:

♦ a belief that back pain is harmful or potentially severely disabling

♦ fear-avoidance behaviour and reduced activity levels

♦ tendency to low mood and withdrawal from social interaction

♦ expectation of passive treatment(s) rather than a belief that active participation will help

---

Figure 1.1 The RCGP guidelines description of yellow flags.

Although there is in reality often little that can be done to alter these factors, a knowledge of them can help lessen frustration when patients fail to respond to treatment in the way expected. More importantly if we GPs can be confident that no one else is going to be in a better position to do more for these patients, then we can be more confident about not referring them for a second opinion. This should help to avoid the miserable cycle of passing them along inappropriately to a specialist, with the ensuing long wait serving to exacerbate the patient's frustration and worries.

In the past many of us may have felt that such a referral was worthwhile because it demonstrated a concern not to leave any stone unturned for our patient and to seek an opinion from a person who we assumed knew more than we did and had more solutions up their sleeve. We also might have felt that we had to refer patients somewhere, to at the very least, share the load of such difficult patients that we hadn't been able to help in our practices.

For a lot of patients, it would be a source of great anger to wait many months to see a surgeon only to be told that surgery would not help and then to be referred back to their GP. Patients would, particularly if the consultation had been brief, often interpret this as callous disregard of their problem and feel deeply affronted. The GP would absorb some of this anger and quite often almost collude with the patient about the disappointing outcome of the appointment because he or she had similarly been hoping for some help!

However enlightened, surgeons do not necessarily feel that they have either the answer or any more wisdom on the subject than their GP colleagues for the majority of patients that come their way and have often been similarly frustrated by having patients in front of them that they cannot help. To manage their time better, they are increasingly using triage physiotherapists to filter their referrals into those suitable for surgery and those with likely serious pathology.[1] The remainder are left in the hands of the physiotherapist or GP.

Does this mean that the GP should be left to cope with these patients unsupported? Of course not! The judicious use of physiotherapy and other physical therapists, such as osteopaths and chiropractors, should help prevent many acute patients becoming chronic and, more importantly, help empower patients to manage their own backs.

Our task is to give clear confident messages about what is realistic and reassure patients that most of them do not need to see a specialist because surgery will not be indicated. We need to tell patients confidently what will help and what will not and to emphasize that more often than not the only people who need to be involved are the patients themselves. It has become a cliché that patients should take responsibility for their own health precisely because it is true and the same applies for their ill-health.

If we give the message that we have a specific solution for recurrent or chronic low back pain then we only have ourselves to blame if we keep seeing the same patient with the same problem. In reality we don't because many patients sense, either from their experience or intuitively, that we cannot help and get on with their lives with greater or lesser amounts of disability.[2] However for some it takes a lot longer to learn this tough lesson, especially for those of a more dependant mentality.

Our challenge therefore is to minimize the disabling affects of low back pain on the lives of our patients. We need to encourage them to manage their symptoms confidently and competently and to give them advice as to how to minimize recurrence and by doing so, help prevent chronicity.

Management in primary care

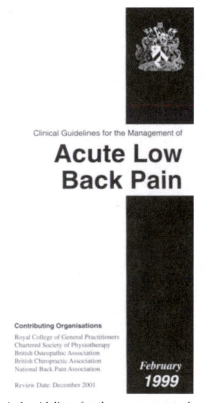

Clinical Guidelines for the Management of

Acute Low Back Pain

Contributing Organisations

Royal College of General Practitioners
Chartered Society of Physiotherapy
British Osteopathic Association
British Chiropractic Association
National Back Pain Association

February
1999

Review Date: December 2001

Figure 1.2 The RCGP clinical guidelines for the management of acute low back pain.

Triage

The first task is to establish whether a patient with low back pain should be principally managed in primary care, the situation in over 90 per cent of cases, or whether secondary care will be needed either urgently, or at a later stage if primary management fails. The RCGP guidelines have started from this initial sorting or triaging, thus providing a good framework from which to consider management. It should be noted that the guidelines refer principally to the first six weeks of management.

> **Diagnostic Triage**
>
> Sort patients into:
>
> - Simple back pain (simple backache);
> - Nerve root pain;
> - Red flags for possible serious spinal pathology;
> - Cauda equina syndrome.

The GP needs to be able to identify which patients may benefit from particular specialist treatment such as surgery and to identify those who might have cancer, an osteoporotic fracture, infection, an inflammatory condition such as ankylosing spondylitis, or who will benefit from other specialist management, such as a functional restoration programme (FRP).

Triage has been drawn from hospital practice rather than from primary care where patient presentations are not always quite so clear-cut as the guidelines make it appear. This is no doubt because the hospital practitioner will have had his patients filtered and sorted to a very large extent by the GP. However the advantage that we have in primary care is that we can triage patients over more than one consultation and in reality patients triage themselves by not attending our surgeries in the majority of episodes of back pain, and by cancelling or not re-attending for follow up consultations.[3]

Triaging for possible serious spinal pathology

Young and older patients have a much higher incidence of serious pathology. In younger patients, particularly those under 20 years of age, there is quite a significant risk of idiopathic deformity or discitis, so these need active consideration and careful undressed examination (see Chapters 9 and 11).

A structural abnormality, such as spondylolisthesis, is similarly commoner in young patients and may be suspected by a history of a feeling of instability volunteered by the patient. Early morning stiffness lasting more than half an hour in the young adult should raise the suspicion of ankylosing spondylitis.

Patients over 55 and possibly even at the age of 50, have a much greater incidence of fractures secondary to osteoporosis or malignancy.[4] A careful history eliciting any pain after minor trauma, sudden unexplained weight loss, general fatigue and malaise, should therefore be sought, together with a careful past history of malignancy from the medical records.

Additionally a previous history of drug abuse, tuberculosis, immuno-suppresion from medication, would serve to alert the doctor to the possibility of infection (see Chapter 9). Thoracic pain in a patient who has not previously had back problems, may be a particularly sinister presentation and merit further investigations. An atypical history, of worsening, unremitting pain, not relieved by rest and which keeps the patient awake at night, may reflect serious underlying pathology.

Symptoms to look out for:

- Sudden, unexplained weight loss;
- Night pain (requiring the patient to get out of bed);
- Night sweats;
- Worsening malaise;
- Recent trauma;
- Worsening deformity;
- Thoracic pain;
- PMH of cancer.

Relevant recent trauma should be elicited and interpreted for that individual. Thus a young fit man who falls onto a pavement outside a pub is much less likely to sustain a fracture than a post-menopausal, frail, elderly lady who might have jarred her back during a bout of coughing or simply coming down the stairs.

Examination will frequently be unrewarding. Screening investigations may require FBC, ESR, CRP, liver function, PSA in older men and a screening MRI scan (if available locally) if malignancy was suspected and/or an urgent referral (see Chapters 12 and 13).

Triaging for nerve root pain

Erudite discussion takes place about the difference between nerve irritation and nerve compression. For the primary care physician this is academic and I will make no attempt to differentiate between the two.

The crucial issue is to identify that nerve root pain may be a possibility by noting from the volunteered history and then asking specifically about any pain, pins and needles or numbness in the legs. Pain predominating in the leg rather than the spine is a good indicator of nerve root pain.

Although satisfying for professional reasons, it is not important to be able to identify precisely where the pathology is in primary care, but just that the problem is nerve root pain as opposed to for example a peripheral neuropathy with its glove-and-stocking bilateral distribution etc.

Once nerve root pain is established, it is important to exclude a cauda equina lesion by ascertaining that there are no significant bowel or urinary symptoms, particularly if the patient has bilateral leg pain. Quite a number of patients will be constipated from a combination of

Table 1.1 Nerve root signs

	Ankle Reflex	*Motor*	*Sensory*
L5	Normal	EHL weakness	Forefoot numbness
S1	TA reflex affected	Calf weakness	Heel numbness

Ninety-eight per cent of nerve root lesions occur at the L5/S1 level.

side-effects of medication and from fear of straining, which will frequently increase any sort of back pain, especially nerve root pain secondary to disc prolapse. In isolation this is not suggestive of cauda equina syndrome and should not deflect from careful questioning about urinary and other bowel disturbances and perianal numbness.

Difficulty passing urine or not having the urge to pass for longer than usual is not a rare symptom in a patient who is in great pain with subsequent high levels of anxiety which may have distracted him or her from even thinking of passing urine. If there are any urinary symptoms, a detailed assessment is needed:

- does the patient feel that they are emptying their bladder completely?
- can he or she feel the urine move along the urethra?
- in the case of a woman, can she tell with confidence that micturition has finished?
- has there been any incontinence of either urine or faeces?
- can the patient differentiate between flatus and motion?
- can the motion be felt passing along through the anus?
- is the bladder extended?

Cauda equina syndrome

- Bilateral leg pain;
- Inability to urinate with extended bladder;
- No sensation of passing urine;
- Saddle anaesthesia;
- Patient unable to distinguish between flatus and motion;
- Progressive motor weakness in the legs or gait disturbance.

The presence of bilateral leg pain is a 'red flag' for cauda equina lesion. However unlikely a cauda equina lesion may seem, even in the presence of good anal tone and peri-anal sensation, it would be a brave (aka foolish) clinician who didn't seek an urgent specialist opinion if there were problems with any of the above.

The next crucial point is whether the straight leg raise (SLR) is reduced. Very slight reduction is common with tight hamstrings, a common finding in sportsmen. However significant reduction of SLR, to usually less than 45 degrees and often less than 30 degrees, is almost pathognomonic of nerve root pain, except in the circumstance of spinal stenosis when the SLR is frequently not affected.

Older patients may present with symptoms of spinal stenosis, i.e. pain in the legs on walking, which are relieved with flexion or sitting (see Chapter 6). In this latter situation there may be a history of nerve root pain coming on after walking which may be eased or settled completely by leaning forwards (e.g. leaning on a supermarket trolley). Differentiation from vascular claudication is usually elicited by asking the

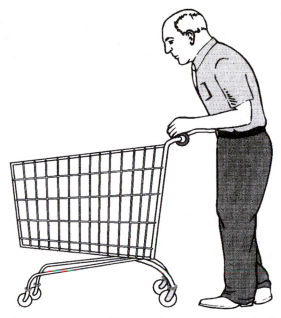

Figure 1.3 Man relieving symptoms of leg pain due to neurogenic claudication by leaning on supermarket trolley.

patient whether flexion reveals the patient's symptoms. Pain that is not relieved by flexion will indicate a vascular cause.

It should be noted that all the possible signs that can be caused by nerve root lesions need not necessarily be present in each case and indeed rarely are although the SLR is the most reliable sign, except for most patients with neurogenic claudication. An absent ankle jerk probably correlates with a more serious lesion than if it is present, but its presence does not rule out a nerve root lesion.

Muscle weakness is the next most likely sign to be present and be particularly likely to be detectable by testing the ankle for dorsiflexion and more specifically looking at the big toe testing extensor hallucis longus. If motor function is significantly impaired the patient may have a dropped foot gait. Sensory changes are not always reliable.

Table 1.2 Differential diagnosis of neurogenic and vascular claudication

	Neurogenic	*Vascular*
Pain on walking	Yes	Yes
Relieved by flexion of spine	Yes	No
Pain on cycling	No	Yes
Pain at rest	Often	No

Management of nerve root pain

The RCGP guidelines suggest that referral for consideration for surgery is unnecessary in most cases within the first four weeks. In practice symptoms often settle later, commonly in the first three months and it is reassuring for patients to be told that there is a very strong likelihood that their symptoms will abate in time, without the need for surgery. If referred for a surgical opinion, in practice, many will have become asymptomatic by the time they are seen anyway.

Patients need to be told what the likely cause of their symptoms is and to be told that no investigations are usually helpful or necessary initially. Reviewing abnormal physical signs, particularly if they revert to normal, give further encouragement but the corollary is that if there are worsening symptoms then urgent referral will be required.

Role of physiotherapy and manipulation in nerve root pain

This is essentially limited to treating any associated back pain and providing reassurance. The evidence to support the use of traction and manipulation is not convincing.

Referral for nerve root pain – neurosurgeon or orthopaedic surgeon?

It is a similar dilemma as to that faced by patients trying to decide between an osteopath and a chiropractor. Essentially most of us cannot judge the performance of particular surgeons as compared to others although this may change.[5] Whoever runs the most patient-centred practice, taking into account waiting times and degree of specialization in back management, would seem reasonable.

Triaging for simple back pain

When the back pain has no obvious cause, the aim should be to confirm, as will be the situation in over 90 per cent of cases, that the pain is mechanical. This means that it will vary in time and place, with clear relieving and exacerbating factors. Any radiation of pain from the back is important, especially if below the knee, when nerve root pain is likely.

Radiation to one or even both buttocks or thighs can occur with mechanical pain but in contrast to nerve root pain will not follow a dermatome, as a rule is rarely worse below the knee and most importantly, is not worse than the actual low back pain.

Simple back pain may be present at rest and when lying in bed. The patient may have difficulty turning in bed. However it will not keep patients awake for long hours during the night or force the patient to get up and sit in a chair. Early morning stiffness is common in patients with simple back pain, but rarely lasts for more than 20 minutes. Simple back pain often worsens as the day progresses, in contrast to the patient with ankylosing spondylitis who improves by the afternoon.

Generally a patient with simple back pain will have been well prior to the onset of their symptoms, although patients will react differently and some will be already dispirited on presentation. A number may present with pre-morbid anxiety and depression, often manifested in poor sleep patterns and general loss of energy and drive. However, sudden unexplained weight loss, combined with severe fatigue should alert one to a possible red flag for malignancy. There should be no significant urinary or bowel symptoms (see Chapter 5).

Simple back pain

- Presentation between ages 20 and 55
- Lumbosacral region, buttocks and thighs
- Pain 'mechanical' in nature
    varies with physical activity
    varies with time
- Patient well
- Prognosis good

There may be little to find. There may be restriction of forward flexion, lateral flexion and rotation. There may be local muscle spasm with palpable tenderness and if severe, a scoliosis. It isn't necessary to do SLR if there is no radiation from the back.[4] However if tested, non-dermatomal referred pain to the leg will not result in a reduced SLR as it may be with true nerve root pain, again, except in the case of neurogenic claudication. Walking may be painful, as often will changing position from sitting to standing. The patient may be in varying degrees of distress.

Management of simple back pain

The most important aspect of management is to give clear confident reassurance about the aetiology and of the expected outcome of a fairly quick recovery. Assuming the worst possible outcome and worrying incessantly about the back problem, are important pre-morbid factors in the genesis of chronic low back pain. It is important to address particular worries and concerns of the patient and dispel any firmly held false beliefs. Avoiding labels like arthritis, with its connotations of chronicity, are important but the most important part of management is to give strong reassurance and confident statements, all of which can be reinforced by a copy of *The Back Book* (see Chapter 3).

If there is no clear precipitant then the cause can frankly be said to be unknown. However, how this is explained can make the difference to a doctor appearing to be hopeless in the patient's eyes or at the cutting edge of low back pain management!

Patients, and hitherto doctors, have been brought up to believe that for proper treatment to be instigated an accurate diagnosis is necessary. Patients understandably crave a precise diagnosis, hoping that it will perforce lead to a logically targeted treatment which will restore the back to its previous healthy state.

This can present quite a challenge. If the patient feels that it is only his GP that cannot tell what is wrong, rather than that it is impossible for any doctor to precisely say where the problem lies, then he may quite reasonably seek a second opinion from another practitioner, be it another doctor, chiropractor or osteopath. He may then be given a very precise diagnosis in manipulative terms which serves to reinforce the notion that the GP did not know much about low back pain.

Since publication of the guidelines, osteopaths and chiropractors have increasingly used the same terminology as ourselves, which has lessened confusion for patients; but some still use a very dramatic sounding engineering model to explain simple back pain and why manipulation works. If manipulation fails, or the patient cannot afford repeated courses of treatment, the different explanations can understandably lead to pressure for a specialist opinion to tell the patient precisely what the problem is.

Managing simple back pain

• Provide reassurance and advice (e.g. *The Back Book*)
• Encourage patients to remain active
• Advise on early return to work if possible
• Refer to physiotherapy or alternative practitioners if no improvement after 2 to 3 weeks

---

Explanation of simple back pain to patients

What do you say simple back pain is to the patient, given that it may have caused anything from minor distress to very great worry and pain? Although a very crucial point in the management, it may seem surprising that there is a dearth of published research on this very issue, so what follows is really a distillation of expert opinions.

It is necessary to emphasize that almost everyone gets back pain to a greater or lesser extent and the normal expected outcome is for it to get better quickly. It can be helpful to explain that anthropologically we were designed to walk on four legs, exercising our bodies far more with less weight coming down onto the lower spine. We now are constantly asking our backs to do something they weren't designed to do such as sitting for long periods in a car or in front of a PC etc. In the course of all this we are bound periodically to put a strain on the ligaments and small joints of the lower spine and pelvis and occasionally the discs in the back.

Additionally it should be pointed out that, poor posture, unsuitable beds, recurrent minor strains from poor lifting techniques may all have led up to a presentation of pain seemingly out of the blue or after minor lifting or twisting. This can be compounded by lack of fitness and aerobic capacity.

The precise problem cannot, and doesn't need, to be pointed out in every patient. It is known that in patients with a history and findings compatible with simple back pain, X-rays and scans won't help. This is because imaging can be very confusing as studies have shown that people with back pain may have normal radiological findings.

In other words, imaging is an unreliable tool for simple back pain and can serve to cause more problems than it solves. However the patient can be reassured that we also know (from extensive research) that because of the very long evolutionary processes that have compensated for a changed role for our bodies, nature is superb at healing itself, given just a little help and no hindrance from ourselves.

One can then list what will help, such as keeping active, taking regular simple analgesics and possibly in the early stages, manipulation or mobilization techniques.

Many patients prefer not to take medication, feeling that they won't know what the state of their back is if they mask it with painkillers. Behind this lies the mistaken belief that if they experience some pain on activity they may be injuring their backs further. This idea needs correcting to enable them to make an informed decision about whether to comply with advice for regular analgesia.

It should be explained that returning to work as soon as practically possible is better than waiting until all pain and stiffness has gone. Resuming early activities such as walking and simple housework, will further aid recovery. It will not damage the back further, provided a modicum of care is taken with regard to lifting and posture. Early activity will most importantly lessen the risks of chronicity and long-term disability. Where heavy lifting is required this is ideally phased back in.

The reason why bed rest is better avoided needs explaining particularly as it is not that long ago that doctors advocated it. Bed rest leads to further deconditioning of the spine and its musculature and reinforces the misconception that the spine is fragile. Additionally it predisposes to deep vein thrombosis.

Referral for physiotherapy

If the back pain has lasted more than a week and the patient has not previously seen a physiotherapist, then referral will help to reinforce the above advice and will provide expert guidance on lifting, back maintenance and exercises. Additionally manipulation, when appropriate, can help and the confidence gained from a skilled professional can have a very positive effect on the patient's morale.

Attending to poor posture, bad ergonomics at work and poor lifting will help prevent many recurrences especially if combined with an improvement in physical fitness, which is often needed.

Physiotherapists can also provide a second opinion of the problem. If the problem is very short-lived and resolves very quickly, then many patients won't wish to see a physiotherapist, but a referral may help to prevent recurrence or lessen their effects. The RCGP guidelines stress the importance of ensuring that resources are made available to facilitate early referral to physiotherapy as the local availability of physiotherapy will influence the timing of such referrals.

Precisely when to refer to a physiotherapist will depend on local facilities, but referral after six weeks with an acute back is known to be less likely to be effective.

Referral for chiropractic or osteopathic treatment

Referral to a chiropractor or osteopath or agreement to that suggestion from a patient, (which is more often the case in practice), may be equally satisfactory. Patients should be encouraged to realize that treatment needs only to be short-term in order to avoid over-reliance on someone other than themselves.

In this respect, knowing the approach of one or two local practitioners may be a worthwhile investment in time to ensure that both parties use the same terminology and agree the same goals. It is thought by some that private practitioners may try to create a dependent patient for financial gain. Given that there is good evidence that manipulation works in acute back pain it is churlish to avoid sensible use of this source of help.

For private practitioners, referrals provide much wanted interaction with mainstream primary care and most will be more than happy to accommodate the above philosophy as their colleges are signed up to the guidelines and indeed contributed to their formation.

Triaging for psychosocial influences

Patients differ greatly in their response to any ill health and this is particularly true of low back pain. Some seem to go into deep decline with worsening disability whilst others appear once in the surgery and never return. Some manage frequent recurrences by seemingly ignoring them and others return repeatedly to a trusted private physiotherapist, chiropractor or osteopath despite the expense.

These observations have been formally acknowledged in the updated 1999 guidelines following research in New Zealand, grouping relevant influences together under the term psychosocial factors.[6]

Disability due to low back pain may be determined by how patients react to illness and injury and how they cope with adversity generally. If people are self-reliant and positive about themselves and life generally, they usually cope with less disability than counterparts who worry greatly and look to others to sort their problems out. Essentially the more frightened patients are, the greater will be the morbidity or disability from the back pain, and the greater the likelihood of chronicity, particularly if they have had prolonged episodes of painful back pain with associated long absence from work.

Additionally, if their life is unsatisfactory either regarding work, marriage or financial problems, their ability to cope with back pain may be diminished. Heavy smoking and alcohol consumption can also have similar effects. Not surprisingly ongoing depression or other health problems further conspire against swift recovery. Previous similar illness behaviour is a further predictor of likely chronicity. Finally, awaiting a specialist appointment, treatment or investigation, has been found to hinder progress.

Premorbid factors that can influence chronic low back pain disability

Dissatisfaction with work
Litigation
Smoking and alcohol consumption
Depression and anxiety
Previous illness behaviour
Waiting times

It is however very important to be clear that this is not to imply that resistant low back pain is all in the mind. It is rather that what is affecting a patient's mind can have a profound effect on his or her disability.

An awareness of the above factors, particularly if progress with an episode is slow, is clearly important and these issues should be addressed as early as possible. Better still is the approach advocated in New Zealand of screening for high risk of chronicity and targeting those patients for extra time and effort, particularly in trying to address their fears and false ideas about the problems that they may have.

Equally important is for the GP not to inadvertently by his or her management increase the risk of chronicity in a patient by, for example, advocating time off work until the episode has completely resolved. Instead, the GP should encourage only the bare minimum of rest and to resume normal activities as soon as possible.

Similarly, an indecent haste to investigate and refer to secondary care, although easy to sympathize with in dealing with patients who sometimes come into the 'heartsink' category, may ultimately be counterproductive. This is despite the considerable pressure for such referrals to be made. Encouragement of self-reliance as outlined in *The Back Book* and taking a generally very positive approach will all help.

Despite all these measures there will inevitably be patients who primarily for psychosocial reasons become chronically disabled and a recognition of this will save frustration for the GP. Additionally it can provide insight into some of the medicolegal disputes the GP may be asked to give evidence for.

The issue of early return to work can cause difficulties when this is perceived to be against both the employee's interests and those of the employer who may have insurance covering sickness absence and only wants his employee back '100 per cent fit'. Inevitably this helps lead to soaring time lost from work through low back pain. Furthermore the employer may feel that he or she is being supportive to their employee when in reality they are conspiring inadvertently to prolong their misery and take the first steps towards long-term disability.

A letter to the employer explaining the best medical interests of the patient might help but unless very carefully phrased might make it sound as if the patient is swinging the lead! A worse problem arises when the patient dislikes their work especially if similar feelings are felt by the employer about the employee. Worse still is the situation when the patient feels that their work has caused their back pain and that continuance of such work might 'wreck their back for good'. One may need to sensitively try to explore these issues with the patient but if compensation is possible, gaining a new job elsewhere is unlikely to happen quickly, if at all, until the claim is resolved.

Encouraging the patient to discuss fears about the effects of his work on his back with their employer who might be prepared to listen if the alternative was costly litigation might help but it is a situation where the GP must not feel disheartened if matters drag on. Facilitation if possible of an ergonomic assessment of the workplace might similarly help although in reality these situations are often beyond the ability of the GP to influence much.

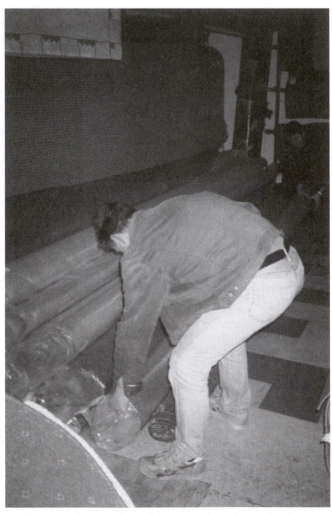

Figure 1.4 Low back pain and the workplace.

Referral to secondary care for chronic low back pain

This may be considered for prolonged or chronically recurrent episodes after due consideration of psychosocial factors as outlined below in this chapter. The first consideration is to clarify with the patient the purpose of the referral. If it is principally to have the benefit of a second opinion on the diagnosis, then this needs to be made clear to the specialist to avoid unnecessary investigations and further appointments. If it is to seek additional help with management then the issue is; to whom should the patient be referred?

A surgeon has the ability to perform a fusion which will help a proportion of patients but make some worse and currently selection for this is somewhat arbitrary, although a large trial is in progress comparing outcomes with a functional restoration programme.[7] However, surgery is not without its risks, which will need to be explained before surgery. If, however, a patient comes away with the belief that he or she may have benefited from the operation, but that it was far too big a risk in his or her case, then this is known to have an adverse effect on back pain disability, so should if possible be avoided (see Chapter 15).

Patients with chronic low back pain mediated by strong psychosocial factors (so called 'Yellow Flags') do not do well with surgery. It will thus be important for the surgeon to be appraised of known psychosocial influences in the referral letter. This may feel uncomfortable for the GP in that it may seem as if he or she is deliberately prejudicing the situation against surgery. However the corollary is of course that to facilitate surgery by omission of relevant facts could lead to inappropriate surgery, to the detriment of the patient. The parallel is that if we fail to mention extensive, serious previous and on-going medical problems, disastrous consequences could befall our patients; so arguably psychosocial factors should be seen in the same light and simply be part of the routinely sent information.

Some evidence suggests that rehabilitation under the auspices of a physician and a team consisting of one or more physiotherapists and clinical psychologists, in what are called functional restoration programmes, may result in better long-term outcomes. Unfortunately these services remain scarce in Britain. If the shift of more resources to primary care does not materialize, as recommended in the RCGP guidelines, then primary care groups and trusts may have to facilitate these programmes themselves.

Summary

A logical simple approach to the management of low back pain in primary care, which takes as its starting point the RCGP guidelines, should result in much greater comfort for both clinician and patient. Confidence is infectious, which coupled with recognition of the importance of psychosocial factors, should result in less morbidity and disability from simple back pain. It should also help patients cope with and manage their back problems more ably. The reader is advised to keep a summary of the guidelines close to hand! Due regard of psychosocial factors should result in better targeted treatment of patients.

References

1. Daker-White Cave, A.J., Harvey, I. *et al.* (1999). A randomised controlled trial. Shifting boundaries of doctors and physiotherapists in orthopaedic out-patient departments. *J. Epidemiol. Community Health*, **53**. 643–650.
2. Croft, P.R., MacFarlane, G.J., Papageorgiou, A.C., Thomas, E. and Silman, A.J. (1998). Outcome of low back pain in general practice: a prospective study. *BMJ*, **316**(7141), 1356–1359.
3. Office for National Statistics Omnibus Survey 1998.
4. Waddell, G. (1998). *The Back Pain Revolution*. Churchill Livingstone.
5. Department of Health UK. (1999). Supporting doctors, protecting patients. A consultation paper on prevention, recognising and dealing with poor clinical performance of doctors in the NHS in England. November 1999. UK Government.
6. ACC. (1997). New Zealand acute low back pain guide. Accident Rehabilitation and Compensation Insurance Corporation of New Zealand and the National Health Committee, Wellington, NZ.
7. Fairbank, J., Frost, H. and Wilson-MacDonald, J. (1994). Proposals for a spinal stabilisation trial. *J. Bone Jt. Surg.*, **76B** (Suppl II–III), 135.

Chapter 2

The Prevalence of Low Back Pain in Great Britain

Paul Pynsent and Mark Webb

Introduction

Back pain is prevalent in the UK with an estimated cost of over £12,000 million to the nation.[1] This prevalence within the general population can be viewed from a number of different perspectives: as a symptom, a cause of disability, a need for health care, or a cause of short or long-term work loss. While a number of recent prevalence estimates have been published from general population surveys in the United Kingdom, comparison of these figures can be problematic[2-4] because of the difficulty in classification.[5] In order to standardize prevalence estimates and then enable comparison between differing surveys, it is important to specify:

(1) Location of pain.
(2) Duration of pain.
(3) Type of standardized questionnaires utilized.

Even with this standardization, symptom recall, non-response rates and unreliable signs[6] remain potential sources of error.

Finally, incidence is defined as the proportion of people in a known population who have presented with the symptom over a particular period of time,[7] that is,

$$\text{Incidence} = \frac{\text{Number of new cases in a period of time}}{\text{Population at risk}}$$

This should be distinguished from prevalence which is the proportion of the population with the disease at a given time, that is,

$$\text{Prevalence} = \frac{\text{Total number of cases at a given time}}{\text{Total population at that time}}$$

Thus it is important to ensure that the parameters for prevalence and incidence have been clearly defined before comparisons are made between studies.

The symptom

Regular surveys have been published on prevalence estimates from the Department of Health. The latest figures for Great Britain are in a

Department of Health bulletin from the Government Statistical Service published 30 June 1999, based on the ONS Omnibus Survey module conducted in March, April and June 1998.[3] Subjects were questioned about back pain experienced within the last year, help sought, advice given, restrictions on activity and time taken off work. Forty per cent of adults report suffering from back pain for more than one day in the previous 12 months. Fifteen per cent experienced back pain throughout the year. There is little difference in the overall prevalence figures for men and women except where age is considered. Females below 24 years and above 65 years of age report more back pain than their male counterparts, however between 45 and 54 years of age males report substantially more pain than women (51 per cent versus 43 per cent, respectively). It is also in this age group that the highest prevalence of back pain is reported for both males and females.

Other recent surveys whose prevalence figures where comparable found similar results, including Dodd[8] who found a prevalence of 40 per cent, Mason[4] who found a prevalence of 37 per cent, Walsh et al.[9] 36 per cent and The South Manchester Study[2] who found a 1 month prevalence of 39 per cent. Reports from North America also show corresponding findings including Von Korrff et al.[10] who found that 41 per cent of American adults aged 26–44 had back pain in the previous 6 months. Surveys in Nordic literature again report similar results – Lebouef-Yde[11] compared a 1992 survey from the general Danish population against four other methodologically similar studies conducted in other Nordic countries between 1977–1985, and demonstrated a prevalence of approximately 50 per cent in over 30-year-olds in the general population.

The current paradigm is that there is an increasing epidemic of low back pain. However, most surveys counter this view and show that the prevalence of low back pain has not changed. Lebouef-Yde (1996)[11] compared figures obtained over a period of almost 20 years and showed significantly consistent prevalence between 1977 and 1995, a further study by the same author in 1995 reviewing 40 years of prevalence figures also supported these findings. The reported differences in prevalence can usually be attributed to the wording of questionnaires, notably the 1 year prevalence of 13.8 per cent in the United States as reported by Deyo and Tsui–Wu.[12] In this survey figures were obtained from the Second National Health and Nutrition Examination Survey which had only included subjects complaining of pain that had lasted for most days within a two-week period. The results of this study could not therefore be compared to the previous studies, which had only utilized data from patients complaining of back pain for more than one day.

In conclusion the evidence provides a cogent argument in support of the view that back pain prevalence remains the same as it has always been.

Disability

Disability does not equal pain and vice versa. Low back pain may impact on general health and well-being, activities of daily living, and work, hence causing disability and handicap – this is very much a social phenomenon. As we have already documented, the apparent epidemic lies at the door of disability and not within low back pain as an isolated symptom. The real change is not in pathology or even in clinical symptoms but in patterns of sick certification and sickness benefits. There has been an increase in chronic disability, medical certification and sickness benefits associated with non-specific low back pain (Figure 2.1). It is important to remember that all surveys give people's own report of their disability – this is naturally purely subjective. Population surveys and official health care statistics will give different results. Only when a claim for sickness benefit or compensation is made is the state able to compile figures. The Department of Social Security (DSS) records benefits paid rather than sickness or work loss and the amount depends on eligibility for benefits. For most workers, sickness lasting up to 28 weeks is now covered by statutory sick pay from their employer and does not appear in DSS statistics, consequently the DSS statistics no longer provide a measure of disability due to back pain.

In Mason's[4] population survey asking respondents about restriction of activity during the four weeks prior to interview, 3 per cent of all adults spent at least one day lying down because of back pain, and 11 per cent of adults said that back pain had restricted their activities in other ways in the preceding 4 weeks. Dodd's[8] reported 8 per cent lying down with 30 per cent saying that they had to restrict their activity and

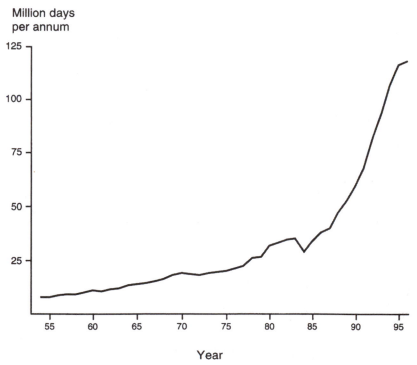

Figure 2.1 UK sickness and invalidity benefits days paid for back pain (based on statistics from the DSS). Adapted with permission from Waddell (1998), p. 2.[14]

Boucher's[3] more recent survey reported that one third of people who reported back pain also had restriction of activity over the preceding four weeks. These reports highlight the gradual increase in the disability caused by back pain as reflected in Figure 2.1. Younger people were less likely than older people to have had restriction (13 per cent of people in the youngest group compared with 40 per cent of people over 65). However there is surprisingly little difference between the ages of 25 and 65. Restriction was mostly reported to normal activities in the home and garden and sporting activities and mobility.

Although pain can cause restriction on social activity, work loss and unemployment due to pain is more worrying. Unfortunately data on this important problem are scanty. Individual employers hold data on actual work loss and consequently there are no national statistics. Mason[4] reported 6 per cent of those aged 16–64 and employed, had taken time off work, Boucher[3] reported similar figures (5 per cent) and Walsh et al.[9] reported a 1 year prevalence of work loss of around 6.5 per cent in women, 9.5 per cent in men. The majority taking less than 7 days off. It is results reported by The Clinical Standards Advisory Group[13] that give the clearest picture to date. They estimated that work loss due to back pain in 1993 was about 52 million days, while 106 million days benefits were paid in respect of back pain. Most of the benefits went to people who were not working anyway and who generally suffer from chronic pain and disability – a now widely accepted fact.

Consultation

What do people do about the pain? In fact, many people with back pain manage it independently most of the time. The South Manchester[2] study reported an annual cumulative incidence in the adult practice populations of 6.4 per cent with 41 per cent of back pain attendees reporting a second consultation within 3 months, while the Fourth National Morbidity Study[8] reported a figure of 8.4 per cent of adults consult in general practice due to back pain and, on average, they have 1.73 consultations. Although back pain is one of the most prevalent symptoms within the general population, it is still not the most common reason for visiting a GP. Respiratory, genitourinary, accidental injuries, skin conditions, infectious diseases and ill-defined signs and symptoms are all still more common reasons for a GP visit. Waddell[14] quotes 4 per cent of all GP consultations in the UK are for back pain.

Despite the prevalence within the population remaining unchanged over the last 40 years, the number seeking advice from their GP with back pain has steadily increased (Figure 2.2). Boucher[3] reported 39 per cent of back pain sufferers consulted their GP in the previous year while Mason[4] reported 16 per cent of adults seeking help from their GP.

Severity of pain naturally governs the need to consult, although the South Manchester Study[2] found little difference between the back pain described by people who sought the opinion of their GP and those who managed it independently. The greatest difference occurred in those

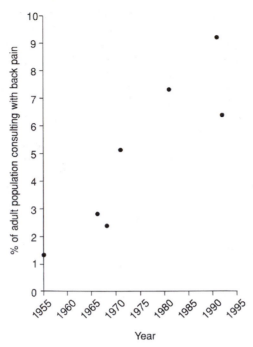

Figure 2.2 Family doctor consultation rates for back pain in the UK. Adapted with permission from Waddell (1998), p. 373.[14]

patients who presented with loss of working hours as a consequence of their back pain. These patients were more likely to seek medical advice, possibly reflecting the need for a sick note. However, what people do about back pain depends as much on the individual as on their medical status. The patient's perception of the problem, their social/emotional status and their individual coping mechanisms will govern whether they seek medical intervention. Patients attending for consultation have differing agendas and needs, whilst still all presenting under the single umbrella of 'low back pain'. Consequently, a variety of issues will need to be addressed, from severity of symptoms to effect on quality of life, from social security benefits and sickness certification to time off work.

Back pain is often not an isolated condition but one constituent of general pain complaints, although the back pain is generally cited as being the most troublesome symptom. Many chronic musculoskeletal pains present as part of a wider clinical picture, including the association between back pain, neck pain and osteoarthritis of the hips and knees. In fact, Badley and Tennant[15] report that in the Calderdale population survey, 23.9 per cent of the population suffered from joint problems with 10.1 per cent affecting the knee, 10 per cent the back and 5.9 per cent the neck. These same patients are also more likely to present with other stress or mental complaints.

Treatment

The vast majority of patients who attend their GP with back pain will receive some form of treatment. Most medical treatment will be passive, including reassurance, advice on rest and prescribed analgesics. In the Mason survey,[4] 64 per cent of patients received medication with approximately a quarter also being advised to have bed rest, and almost a quarter were given a sick note. A fifth of GP consultations were referred to hospital for advice on management, for reassurance of the patient and GP, to establish a diagnosis or to take over treatment. The South Manchester Study showed the duration of back pain in 91 per cent of these patients to be greater than 3 months in the last year, with 73 per cent having continuous pain.

Most patients attending hospital have chronic low back pain and are not working, typically they have already been referred on more than one occasion with a similar symptom or diagnosis. These patients have higher disability and are more resistant to improvement than acute sufferers.[16] Again the South Manchester Study interviewed patients 3 months after their outpatient visit and most said they had no change in their condition, in fact 91 per cent still had back pain.

Summary

- About 35–40% of adults have back pain within a one year time span.
- About 5–10% report some low back disability within one year.
- There is no evidence of any change in low back pain pathology.
- The prevalence of low back pain has not changed.
- There is an exponential rise in chronic disability, medical certification and sickness benefit.
- Four per cent of all GP consultations are for back pain.

References

1. Maniadakis, N. and Gray, A. (2000).The economic burden of back pain in the UK. *Pain*, **84**, 95–103.
2. Papageorgiou, A.C., Croft, P.R., Ferry, S., Jayson, M.I.V. and Silman, A.J. (1995). Estimating the prevalence of low back pain in the general population. Evidence from the South Manchester back pain survey. *Spine*, **20**, 1889–1894.
3. Boucher, A. (1999). *The prevalence of back pain in Great Britain in 1998*. ONS Omnibus Survey. Office of National Statistics, HMSO.
4. Mason, V. (1994). *The prevalence of back pain in Great Britain*. Office of Population Censuses and Surveys, Social Survey Division. pp. 1–24. HMSO.
5. Pynsent, P.B. and Fairbank, J.C.T. (1990) Back pain – a hierarchical nosology. In *Back Pain. Classification of Syndromes* (J.C.T. Fairbank and P.B. Pynsent eds), Manchester University Press.
6. McCombe, P.F., Fairbank, J.C.T., Cockersole, B.C. and Pynsent, P.B. (1989). Reproducibility of physical signs in low-back pain. *Spine*, **14**, 906–918.
7. Armitage, P. and Berry, G. (1987). *Statistical Methods in Medical Research*. Blackwell Scientific.

8. Dodd, T. (1996). *The Prevalence of Back Pain in Great Britain in 1996*. Office of Population Censuses and Surveys, Social Survey Division. HMSO.

9. Walsh, K., Cruddas, M. and Coggon, D. (1992). Low back pain in eight areas of Britain. *J. Epidemiol. Community Health*, **46**, 227–230.

10. Von Korff, M., Dworkin, S.F., Le Resche, L. and Kruger, A. (1988). The epidemiologic comparison of pain complaints. *Pain*, **32**, 173–183.

11. Lebouef –Yde, C., Klougart, N., Mauritzen, T. (1996). How common is low back pain in the Nordic population? Data from a recent study on a middle aged general Danish population and four surveys previously conducted in the Nordic Countries. *Spine*, **21**, 1518–1525.

12. Deyo, R.A. and Tsui-Wu, Y.-J. (1987). Functional disability due to back pain. *Arthritis and Rheumatism*, **30**, 1247–1253.

13. Clinical Standards Advisory Group. (1994). *Epidemiology Review: The Epidemiology and Cost of Back Pain. Annex to CSAG Report on Back Pain*. pp. 1–72. HMSO.

14. Waddell, G. (1998). The epidemiology of low back pain. In *The Back Pain Revolution* (G. Waddell, ed.), Churchill Livingstone.

15. Badley, E.M. and Tennant, A. (1992). Changing profile of joint disorders with age: findings from a postal survey of the population of Calderdale, West Yorkshire, United Kingdom. *Ann. Rheumat. Dis.*, **51**, 366–371.

16. Fairbank, J.C.T. and Pynsent, P.B. (2000). The Oswestry Disability Index. *Spine*, (in press).

Simple Back Pain

Chapter 3

Simple Back Pain

Richard Bartley

Low back pain in the 21st Century remains an ubiquitous problem. It is an important reason for work absence, rising social security payments and considerable distress for sufferers, not just in the United Kingdom, but across the industrialized world.[1] Eighty per cent of people in Britain develop back pain at some point.[2] Ninety per cent improve by 12 weeks.[3] The remaining 10 per cent have persistent chronic pain lasting three months or longer and account for considerable social costs.[4]

Despite its universal prevalence, only 2 per cent of patients reporting low back pain are found to have a serious cause, of which roughly half are rheumatic, the remainder consisting of serious spinal diseases such as tumours and infections. Only 5 per cent of low back pain patients present with true nerve root pain. The remaining 93 per cent of the low back population experience mechanical pain of musculoskeletal origin, so called simple back pain.[4]

Table 3.1 Sub-classification of low back pain

Simple back pain	93%
Nerve root pain	5%
Suspected serious pathology	2%
Inflammatory	1%
Tumours, infections etc.	1%

Pathology

Waddell states that definite pathology can only be diagnosed in 15 per cent of patients reporting low back pain.[4] Many attempts have been made in the past to sub-classify low back pain, often on pathoanatomical grounds, but usually without any consensus on agreement of terminology or diagnostic criteria between different researchers and clinicians.[5] The numerous pain-sensitive structures in the lumbosacral spine cause common symptoms and presentation and therefore diagnoses based on identifying individual anatomical structures in the spine invariably fail.

Commonly identified features such as limitation of spinal movements, radiological spondylosis, facet joint osteoarthritis or disc degeneration and protrusion identified on magnetic resonance imaging only correlate weakly with the presence of back pain.[6] Epidemiological studies have demonstrated little or no correlation between back pain and inherited factors, such as height, weight, deformity (unless gross), spinal movements, gross muscle strength, or radiological signs of disc degeneration.[7] Recent MRI studies, however, suggest that there may be some correlation between early degenerative disease of the lumbar discs in young people being predictors of low back pain in later life.[8,9] Of much more importance are smoking, psychological morbidity, poor work conditions, social class, education and income.

It is not possible to identify individual structures, such as intervertebral discs, facet or sacro-iliac joints, as independent causes of low back pain. Clinical tests for these lack sensitivity and specificity. Scans, such as MRI, can identify time-related changes in tissue architecture but cannot identify painful structures.[10] Whilst provocative tests, such as discograms and joint blocks, can elicit the presence or absence of pain mediators within an individual structure, they cannot take into account the complexity of anatomical interaction, particularly when these structures are loaded. For example, a painful facet joint confirmed by a diagnostic facet block does not exclude the presence of other pain sources in the spine and the use of therapeutic blocks may therefore not guarantee the relief of pain.

Labelling simple back pain patients with diagnoses such as lumbar spondylosis, arthritis, sacro-iliac lesions, facet joint lesions and 'slipped discs' have little clinical relevance and only serve to reinforce the patient's notion that he/she has incurred irreversible damage which can only be confirmed by expensive imaging studies. Until clinical and radiological tests have greater sensitivity and specificity, the validity of current sub-classifications of simple low back pain, commonly used by healthcare practitioners today, are better avoided.

Features

In contrast to earlier unsatisfactory attempts to sub-classify simple back pain based on purely anatomical clinical syndromes, the RCGP guidelines provide simple criteria to assist the clinician in differentiating simple back pain from more serious causes such as nerve root pain and possible serious pathology.

These are:

- the patient is aged between 20 to 55;
- the patient is well;
- the pain is felt in the lumbosacral area, buttocks and thighs;
- the pain is mechanical in nature, i.e. it varies with activity and time.

Age

The commonest age range for patients reporting low back pain to their GP is 45 to 59,[3] but back pain can be reported at any age, including patients aged under 20 and over 55. However pain reported in these latter age groups should make the clinician especially vigilant to exclude specific causes for low back pain that are peculiar to that particular age group. Examples include discitis in children and osteoporotic fractures in older patients.

Constitutional status

Patients with simple back pain report normal health, unless a known concomitant illness is occurring independently of the acute low back pain. Constitutional symptoms such as recent unexplained weight loss, unremitting pain not relieved by activity or rest, night sweats and worsening malaise should always raise the level of suspicion.

Site of pain

According to Nachmeson,[11] the definition of low back pain refers to pain felt in the area extending from the lower rib cage to the gluteal folds. However, many clinicians would also include thigh pain. As a definition, low back pain does not include pain below the knee or far lateral to the midline of the lumbar spine (which is described as loin pain and may in some cases indicate pain of a visceral origin).

Patients with simple back pain frequently report 'referred' pain in the buttocks and thighs. This is not the same as radicular pain (or true sciatica) which is a manifestation of a nerve root lesion. Referred pain usually has a vague distribution in the leg and is not reproduced by the straight leg raise test or femoral stretch test (see Chapter 5).

More importantly, the patient with nerve root pain will almost always report that their leg pain is worse than any back pain they may have. This is not the case for patients with simple low back pain who invariably stress that their back pain is the worst site of pain. It can be useful to ask the patient – "which would they prefer to be treated?".

The mechanical nature of simple back pain

Mechanical low back pain is sensitive to changes in posture and activity. However not all patients will necessarily report pain with activity and improvement with rest. Patients frequently report that prolonged sitting or lying can make their pain worse and that sometimes sustained activity helps. The important point is that there are clear exacerbating and relieving factors.

Very occasionally, patients with serious underlying pathology will present with what appears to be 'mechanical' pain in the early stages of the disease (Grieve described these as 'masqueraders'[12]). However their symptoms often progress rapidly and do not respond to conventional treatment. A failure to improve with time and conservative care should alert the clinician to a potential red flag.

Prognosis

Ninety per cent of patients with simple back pain appear to improve within 12 weeks of onset. However many will continue to experience some symptoms. The South Manchester study in 1997 identified that up to 83 per cent of patients will still report on-going symptoms up to 12 months after the initial episode.[3] Acute and chronic definitions can be therefore misleading. Patients presenting to their GP with acute low back pain are often likely to be experiencing an 'acute-on-chronic' episode.

Patients reporting simple back pain typically experience one or more episodes of acute pain with periods of remission, characterized by mild or no backache. Sometimes these episodes become more frequent with a gradual deterioration in the healing time. Although this does not necessarily mean that the patient is re-injuring the same soft tissue structures within the spinal column, it may reflect a deterioration in lumbopelvic muscle tone and co-ordination that can result from an initial injury.[13,14]

A few patients may eventually fall out of the job market following a long history of acute low back pain episodes. Some of these patients may be offered surgery in the form of a spinal fusion. Whilst a number of fusion techniques exist, the efficacy of spinal surgery for patients with recurrent acute low back pain remains very much open to question (see Chapter 15).

Gibson *et al.* in a systematic review in 1999, concluded that 'there was no scientific evidence about the effectiveness of any form of [surgical fusion] for degenerative lumbar spondylosis compared with natural history, placebo or conservative treatment'.[15]

Psychosocial risk factors

The majority of patients with recurrent acute low back pain do not become disabled and it could be argued that recurring low back pain is a normal human experience.[4] However some patients have continuous low back pain lasting more than three months, causing considerable disability and these can be classed as having chronic low back pain.

The Clinical Standards Advisory Group (CSAG) report on low back pain in Great Britain in 1994 referred to 'psychosocial' back pain and stressed that non-organic factors may be as important as physical causes in the genesis of chronic low back pain disability.[16] Idiosyncratic social and cultural attitudes to disease and ill-health frequently determine individuals response to low back pain.[4] These can be compounded by the availability of social security payments and disability allowances and whether potential recipients qualify for them. Personal and family beliefs add to this complicated picture.

The New Zealand clinical guidelines on low back pain in 1998 stressed that psychosocial factors are not simply responses to pain. They are in fact important predictors of chronicity. They can determine how patients will respond to injury, what healthcare they will seek and how they will respond to medical and therapeutic intervention. They will also determine whether they will request time off work (some indefinitely) and whether they will pursue litigation.

These views are supported by the South Manchester studies on low back pain which identified pre-morbid psychosocial factors as important predictors of long-term low back pain disability.[17] They found that poor work satisfaction, psychological distress, smoking and duration of symptoms all contributed to chronic low back pain. Pursuing legal claims can also greatly influence outcomes.

It is now recognized that psychosocial factors can manifest themselves in the first few days or weeks following the onset of the patient's symptoms and the New Zealand guidelines stress the importance of recognizing these signs early so that appropriate healthcare can be implemented as soon as possible to minimize long-term disability. The guidelines identified these psychosocial risk factors as 'Yellow Flags'[18] and require the GP or triage clinician to be as vigilant of them as the physical risk factors, i.e. 'Red Flags'.

Yellow Flags	Red Flags
Psychosocial risk factors	Physical risk factors
Chronic illness behaviour	Possible serious pathology

Early signs of psychosocial low back pain are:

- a wide symptom pattern of worsening low back pain and referred pain to the lower limbs, which is frequently associated with neck pain and non-dermatomal sensory changes on one side of the body or all four limbs;
- hypersensitivity to normal sensory stimuli;
- disturbed sleep patterns;
- avoidance of work and social interaction;
- the presence of 'Waddell signs'; positive responses to clinical tests that are designed to differentiate organic and non-organic signs[4] (Table 3.2).

These factors can be influenced by an overprotective, or conversely an unsupportive, spouse or family network and medical attendant.

Table 3.2 Waddell signs

1. Tenderness that is either superficial or non-anatomic in distribution or both.
2. Simulation of back pain stimulation by axial loading (pressure on the vertex of the erect subject or rotation of the pelvis and shoulders in the same plane avoiding spinal movement).
3. Discrepancies in 'straight leg raising test' performance in the sitting and supine positions.
4. Regional disturbance such as stocking distribution of hyperaesthesia or generalized weakness of a region.

Physical symptoms and signs which, when combined, point to the presence of non-organic factors in the production of back pain (Waddell signs). Adapted with permission from Waddell (1998), p. 162.[4]

A further complication can be the difficulty in providing the patients with an exact diagnosis in the acute stage of their low back pain. This can be frustrating both to the patient and the clinician and may be another important non-organic mediator of chronic low back pain, with the patient often opting to 'shoot the messenger' rather than accept the facts. It invariably leads patients to 'shop around' eventually arriving at the doorsteps of less circumspect practitioners who may be more willing to provide them with a 'diagnosis', however fanciful it turns out to be.

Who is to blame for rising low back pain disability?

The case for iatrogenic chronic low back pain is a contentious one. Some observers lay the root causes of rising low back pain disability and spiralling social security costs at the doors of the medical profession and the social security system. They argue that low back pain has become over-medicalized and that this is leading to unacceptable levels of disability that do not exist in the under-developed world.[4]

Contributing factors to an epidemic of low back pain disability in the UK include:

- poor medical advice (e.g. advocating bed rest for acute low back pain) and pain management;
- a failure to separate the GP's responsibility for the clinical management of low back pain from determining eligibility for disability allowance;
- non-evidence based practice carried out by many misguided practitioners who create dependency in the back pain population on these professions.

These iatrogenic factors go hand-in-hand with modern late 20th century lifestyles. British society is not unique in having increased leisure time and labour saving gadgets both in the workplace and in the home. Levels of obesity and poor general fitness levels continue to rise and this is associated with an increase in the incidence of non-insulin-dependent diabetes mellitus, heart and bowel disease and other chronic maladies.[19]

Smoking is recognized by a number of high quality studies to influence the incidence of low back pain (although a recent review suggested the link between smoking and low back pain may not be as strong as previously thought,[20] other studies continue to stress that smoking can exacerbate low back pain.[21]).

There is good evidence that the more the patient participates in his or her own healthcare the better the chance of making a speedy recovery.[22] Many patients have out-dated expectations of a 'cure' or that the only effective remedies are those that involve their passive participation, whether it involves surgery or palliative physical therapy in the form of heat and electrical treatments.

Unfortunately too many back care providers are often too willing to collude with these outdated expectations, however well-meaning their intentions, although it should be stressed that many do not. This can be a particularly difficult problem in the private sector where business needs driven by consumer satisfaction can make it difficult for practitioners to deliver evidence-based healthcare.

Evidence-based practice

A plethora of treatments are available for simple back pain, nearly all of which are non-evidence-based. Surgeons are as guilty of this as any of the conservative remedies used by physical therapists. Radiological interventions, such as therapeutic facet blocks, lack any scientific basis for their efficacy.

A consumer-led approach places pressure on GPs and other clinicians to provide these treatments. However even the most hardened advocate of evidence-based practice would agree that these empirical treatments continue to have a place, provided both clinicians and patients are aware of their limitations. It must be recognized that they should be used with the explicit aim of enabling the patient to rehabilitate himself and return to normal activities and work as soon as possible.

Where non-evidence-based practice is potentially harmful is when it fails to involve the patient's active participation, both in terms of prevention of injury and disease, and in response to them. The lack of understanding by some clinicians of the importance of evidence-based practice continues to undermine the efforts of those attempting to improve the system of managing patients with low back pain.

Pain and disability

The advocates of the psychosocial model of low back pain have made an important contribution to the debate on how low back pain should be managed in the UK and other industrialized countries. For too long both patients and clinicians have failed to recognize that pain and disability

---

The World Health Organisation (WHO) Model of Impairment, Disability and Handicap.[23]

Disability can be viewed as part of a continuum:

PATHOLOGY ..... IMPAIRMENT ...... DISABILITY ..... HANDICAP

Pathology may lead to impairment, e.g. a painful back, a swollen stiff knee.

Disability is restricted function (WHO, 1988). It is the practical consequences of having one or more impairments, e.g. the inability to walk to the shops due to neurogenic claudication. Observing disability in patients enables clinicians to observe the impact of the disease without ignoring other important factors that may influence the patient, e.g. attitudes to pain tolerance, social and economic circumstances.

Handicap is the social consequences of the patient's disability, e.g. the patient with neurogenic claudication unable to collect his pension.

are not interdependent. In other words, lumbosacral pain may have a physical cause (usually self-limiting), but it is the patient's response to this pain that determines reported levels of disability.

Patients may experience significant impairment and pain without significant disability, in other words, they continue to lead normal lives despite their pain. However the reverse is also true. Levels of disability in the United Kingdom due to back pain appear to be rising in the absence of evidence that back pain is any more prevalent today than since the introduction of the British welfare state 50 years ago.

Waddell (1987) described disability as the most important measure among low back pain disorders, rather than pain.[24] The effective management of the patient with acute low back pain can prevent chronicity and unnecessary disability.[25] The New Zealand guidelines stressed the importance of early detection and appropriate management of potential chronic low back pain patients to prevent disability. This all points to a change in emphasis from simply providing healthcare in response to pain to addressing low back pain disability and its causes.

The disability model approach requires a radical change in how low back pain patients are managed. A new paradigm is needed, one which incorporates effective early triage and evidence-based treatment regimes.

Diagnostic triage

Diagnostic triage should form the basic approach to managing patients with low back pain. Patients should be assessed and examined, as described in Table 3.3, and prioritized according to surgical or medical need.

The aim of triage is to exclude non-mechanical causes, provide appropriate treatment and avoid unnecessary costly investigation. It should be possible to categorize the patient into one of the following groups:

- simple back pain;
- nerve root pain;
- spinal pathology including tumour, infection, bone disease, primary neurological disease and inflammatory conditions, such as ankylosing spondylitis;
- cauda equina syndrome.

Warning signs to suggest the need for further evaluation to exclude suspected serious pathology as listed in the guidelines are:

- constant unremitting pain and pain that is not affected by movement;
- generalized bone pain;
- age over 55 years – they may have osteoporosis but also have a higher risk of secondary malignancy or myeloma;
- focal neurological symptoms and signs of cauda equina syndrome; leg pain dominating back pain and associated with objective physical signs (if it correlates with findings on imaging surgical decompression is likely to be beneficial);

Table 3.3 Assessment and examination of the patient

Assessment of the patient

History
- current symptoms
- exacerbating and relieving factors
- night pain
- diurnal pattern
- early morning stiffness

Previous medical history
- general health
- current medication
- previous back pain

Special questions
- history of RA, steroid use
- bladder/bowel disturbances
- neurological symptoms
- cough impulse sign for leg pain

Investigations
- bloods
- plain X-rays
- CT/bone scan/MRI/Dexa

Examination of the patient

Observation
- performance (e.g. getting undressed)
- deformity (local or global)
- changes in muscle tone
- swelling
- gait
- spine ranges of movement
- hip joint

Neurological tests
- straight leg raise/ femoral stretch test
- reflexes, sensation, motor power & tone
- plantar responses
- proprioception and co-ordination (if indicated)

Palpation
- spine (look for marked tenderness)
- abdomen (look for masses)

- pain worse on walking downhill relieved by a few minutes sitting and better on going uphill (lumbar flexion) suggests neurogenic claudication;
- systemic illness and night sweats (TB classically affects the upper lumbar and lower thoracic vertebrae);
- early morning stiffness better with exercise – suggestive of ankylosing spondylitis;
- thoracic pain is much less common than lumbar or cervical pain and requires further evaluation;
- those with a previous history of cancer;
- those under 25 years e.g. spondylolisthesis, scoliosis.

Sources of referred pain to the spine

Hip joint
Aortic aneurysm
Aortic dissection
Renal disease
Gynaecological pain
Pelvic tumour
Pancreatic and other retroperitoneal disease

Leg pain, if worse than lumbosacral pain, should lead the clinician to suspect nerve root lesion. This also includes patients whose walking tolerance is greatly reduced by leg pain.

All other cases fall into the category of simple back pain and should usually be managed in the community.

It should be noted that not all patients will fit neatly into one of the three sub-groups of low back pain. Some patients may present with what seems to be reasonable signs of simple back pain, but with one or two slightly unusual symptoms.

The GP needs to further investigate what the patient means by reported symptoms, for example night pain. If the pain is not sufficient to encourage the patient to leave his bed this probably implies that the pain is still mechanical, i.e. it is posturally related. Pain that forces the patient out of bed suggests intractable pain that requires further investigation.

Plain X-rays cannot be used to diagnose simple back pain and have poor sensitivity for serious pathology.[4] One study suggests that routine plain X-rays of the lumbar spine contributes to up to 19 deaths a year in the UK.[26] Their routine use in the management of acute low back pain is discouraged by the Royal College of Radiologists.

Royal College of Radiologists recommendations

- There is no indication for routine X-rays in acute LBP of less than 6 weeks in the absence of clinical red flags.
- Unnecessary or repeated X-rays should be avoided.
- Lumbar spine X-rays involve 150 times the radiation dose of a chest X-ray.

Simple laboratory investigations such as full blood count, ESR and C-reactive protein may detect sinister pathology and are sensitive to some, but not all, rheumatic conditions such as polymyalgia rheumatica. However these are non-specific tests and should only be used to complement clinical findings (i.e. any identified 'Red Flags').[4] Prostatic specific antigen (PSA) is a useful screen for male patients over 55 years of age with severe, intractable low back pain (a prostate examination may also be necessary). Alkaline phosphatase is a useful screen for malignancy.

Whilst the GP is always under pressure not to over-investigate patients, it is argued by some clinicians that a low index for investigating unusual symptoms is a reflection of safe medical practice. If the investigations are normal and the clinical presentation suggests simple back pain, the patient and the GP will then be able to pursue a more conservative physical therapy approach to dealing with the patient's symptoms.

However this view is contested fiercely by others who see the use of expensive imaging as an unnecessary waste of healthcare resources and which only reinforce the unrealistic expectations of patients seeking a gold standard diagnosis and cure. Can the discovery of one case of a dissecting aneurysm or a benign primary tumour per 1000 screening MR scans be justified?

The introduction of low-cost limited-study MR investigations, used instead of plain X-rays, for *some* patients may appear as a compromise to many clinicians. However such a facility is not yet universally available (see Chapter 12).

A model for managing simple back pain

It is not necessary for patients with simple back pain to be referred to a consultant orthopaedic surgeon, unless there is some perceived evidence of instability. A team-based approach, co-ordinated by the GP, with physical therapists and nurse providing expertise and support, should suffice for the management of the great majority of these patients.

The requirements for effective management of patients with low back pain involves a change in the way services are run within primary care and a cultural shift within the whole healthcare community, including the private sector.

The system of healthcare in the United Kingdom has undergone a number of reforms since the NHS began in 1948. The latest of these has healthcare purchasers divided into primary care groups (PCGs) and, more recently, primary care trusts (PCTs).

These organizations need to encourage a shift of resources from secondary to primary care in order to provide:

● up-to-date training for healthcare professionals;
● enhanced physiotherapy support for GPs;
● community-based specialist services for patients with chronic back pain;
● educational materials, such as *The Back Book*.

A shift in resources from secondary care to primary care may not be easy to bring about. It could be anticipated that hospital-based clinicians would not wish to see their resources reduced even further. However additional resources in primary care are essential if the management of low back pain and other chronic conditions are to be managed more efficiently.

Imaging

Purchasers should also develop better support services for GPs, particularly in radiology, where the judicious use of direct access to limited (and less costly) MRI could improve the management of some patients with low back pain.

Chronic pain management

Dedicated services for patients with chronic low back pain would also greatly assist the GP. This is discussed in Chapter 4.

Such dedicated services currently exist in Britain and typically involve a multi-professional team, consisting of a physician, anaesthetist or GP, one or two physiotherapists, a nurse and a clinical psychologist. The team is responsible for developing rehabilitation programmes for these patients, which are often described as functional restoration programmes (FRPs). Some evidence exists to support the use of FRPs.[27]

Unfortunately, these services are scarce in the British Isles, leaving GPs with the burden of managing these complex patients. It seems curious that healthcare purchasers seem willing to purchase expensive surgery for patients with low back pain yet are often unwilling to purchase FRPs, both approaches equally supported by only a moderate amount of supporting evidence for their use. This again reflects an intransigent healthcare culture that is all too often led by hospital-based services at the expense of primary healthcare providers. It is ultimately the responsibility of GPs to change the status quo, although nobody would expect this to be an easy task.

Triage physiotherapists

GPs can also be greatly assisted by suitably trained physiotherapists. Many of these clinicians have excellent triage skills that are put to use by

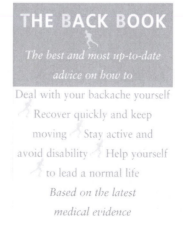

Figure 3.1 The Back Book.

GPs. A number of successful schemes have already proved to be cost-effective in a number of hospitals across the United Kingdom, and new physiotherapy-led triage services are developing in primary care (see Chapter 17).

Patient information

A useful tool for the busy GP is *The Back Book*, issued by the HMSO in Great Britain. *The Back Book* carries prominent messages about self-reliance and the need to remain active following an acute episode of low back pain. Burton et al., in 1998, found that patients respond positively to the book.[28,29]

Timing

Time is critical in the effective management of simple back pain. Early and effective intervention, which need not necessarily involve referral to another healthcare professional, can help prevent disability and subsequent costs to the healthcare system, as well as the GP's mental well-being!

Treatment responses must be appropriate to the length of time the patent has experienced low back pain, his beliefs about illness and pain, and his expectations of healthcare. Very acute low back pain may need little intervention by the GP. Indeed, many people experiencing low back pain do not seek healthcare at all.[3]

Providing simple information in the early stage of a back pain episode may be as effective as a traditional course of physiotherapy or chiropractic intervention. Emphasis on resuming normal daily activities and discouraging bed rest is very important.[30] Young in 1995 demonstrated that one-off advice sessions to be as effective as traditional physiotherapy and chiropractic for sufferers of acute low back pain.[25] This approach reduced costs and encouraged patients to be self-reliant.

Guidelines for the management of acute low back pain

1. Drug management should involve the use of simple analgesia with use of NSAIDS if necessary. Opiate-based drugs should be avoided. The use of muscle relaxants may be indicated in a few patients but their widespread use is not supported by current medical literature.
2. Discourage bed rest. Bed rest should not be used as a treatment, although one or two days may be necessary for a patient in considerable pain. Prolonged bed rest raises the risk of deep vein thrombosis and can lead to considerable stiffness and deconditioning of the spine.
3. Encourage return to early activities and work is also recommended. The patient's pain may not necessarily be worse if she or she returns to work, unless the job involves heavy manual work.

4. Avoid routine X-ray examination of patients with low back pain (as recommended by the Royal College of Radiologists).
5. Above all, refrain from suggesting a physical explanation for the patent's symptoms as this is difficult to confirm clinically and only serves to reinforce the notion that the patient has something significantly wrong with him.

Patients who fail to improve after two weeks may respond to physical therapy intervention (i.e. physiotherapy, chiropractic or osteopathy). Developing a close working relationship with any of these practitioners can help the GP to manage these patients. If NHS resources are not available to support local physiotherapy services, patients could be encouraged to seek the assistance of private practitioners (many will provide concessions to low income patients). Some PCGs already have successful contracts with non-NHS services. Agreed protocols between these professionals and the GP can help to encourage the use of evidence-based practice and common language to avoid confusing patients with mixed messages and diagnoses.

Some patients may need fitness re-training if they have been off work for two or more weeks, or muscular weakness and general de-conditioning of the spine have been identified. This can involve twice-weekly aerobic exercise classes, combined with advice and specific muscle reconditioning exercises. This approach has been the subject of a number of studies which have demonstrated its effectiveness.[31,32] These programmes are suitable for patients who have improved following an episode of acute low back pain, who need to return to full fitness. They may not be suitable for patients who show no signs of improvement.

In this case, patients who fail to improve after six weeks should prompt the GP or physical therapist to consider whether the patient presents with

Table 3.4 A timetable for managing acute low back pain

DURING FIRST WEEK AFTER THE ONSET OF THE PAIN	General practitioner or practice physical therapist to perform diagnostic triage. For simple low back pain prescribe moderate analgesia and NSAIDs and give advice and reassurance. *The Back Book* (ISBN 011 702 0788) provides simple, straightforward advice for patients.
IF NO IMPROVEMENT AFTER TWO WEEKS	Refer to chiropractor, osteopath or physiotherapist for assessment and treatment e.g. manipulation (UK patients should be encouraged to use non-NHS practitioners if local resources do not allow rapid access to NHS physiotherapy. NHS providers should consider purchasing services from local non-NHS providers).
IF NO IMPROVEMENT AFTER 6 WEEKS OF PHYSICAL TREATMENT	Reassessment of the patient. Assess for red or yellow flags. Refer to appropriate specialist if these are present; otherwise patient should undergo rehabilitation or aerobic reconditioning.

'red' or 'yellow' flag symptoms and signs. However it could be argued that such vigilance is necessary from the time of the patient's first contact with either the GP or physiotherapist. The earlier either of these two subgroups are detected the better the prognosis.

Patients with 'red' flag symptoms and signs should be referred to an orthopaedic or neurosurgical consultant. 'Yellow' flag patients should be referred to a specialist chronic pain service. This is discussed in the next chapter.

A useful algorithm is shown in Table 3.4.

Summary

The management of simple back pain can be summarized as follows:

When assessing the patient

1. Recognize the importance of psychosocial factors.
2. Avoid making clinical decisions purely on biomedical grounds.
3. Encourage early return to work, maintenance of normal daily activities, avoidance of bed rest.
4. Discourage 'techno fix' treatments and investigations.
5. Provide educational materials for patients.

Additional support

1. Make use of specialist physical therapist with training in diagnostic triage.
2. Only refer to hospital specialist if the patient presents with 'red flag' signs.
3. Put pressure on health purchasers to fund a chronic pain service if one does not already exist.

If in doubt

1. Take ESR & FBC.
2. Arrange direct access to limited study magnetic resonance imaging or conventional imaging, but do not routinely X-ray patients.

Overall management

1. Encourage a primary-care team approach where:
   - the GP takes the lead and ultimate responsibility for the patient;
   - physical therapists and nurses provide expertise and support;
   - communication is improved, so that healthcare professionals 'speak the same language' when dealing with patients.
2. Encourage shared responsibility so that patients:
   - accept that they have duties as well as rights;

- are realistic about treatment aims;
- recognize that there are limited resources and that they may need to accept some financial responsibilities when services may be unavailable.
3. Encourage physical therapists to:
  - practice evidence-based medicine.
  - encourage patient responsibility and make moderate use of passive interventions;
  - avoid 'labelling' or dressing up theories as facts;
  - provide rehabilitation for patients with recurrent or chronic low back pain.

References

1. Bigos, S.J., Battie, M.C., Spengler, D.M., Fisher, L.D., Fordyce, W.E., Hansson, T., Nachemson, A.L. and Zeh, J. (1992). A longitudinal, prospective study of industrial back injury reporting. *Clin. Orthop.*, **279**, 21–34.
2. Macfarlane, G.J., Thomas, E., Croft, P.R., Papageorgiou, A.C., Jayson, M.I. and Silman, A.J. (1999). Predictors of early improvement in low back pain amongst consulters to general practice: the influence of pre-morbid and episode related factors. *Pain*, **80**(1–2), 113–119.
3. Croft, P.R., MacFarlane, G.J., Papageorgiou, A.C., Thomas, E. and Silman, A.J. (1999). Outcome of low back pain in general practice: a prospective study. *BMJ*, **316**(7141), 1356–1359.
4. Waddell, G. (1998). *The Back Pain Revolution*. Churchill Livingstone.
5. Fairbank, J.C.T. and Pynsent, P.B. (1990). *Back Pain. Classification of Syndromes*. Manchester University Press.
6. Boos, N., Riedr, R., Schader, V. *et al.* (1995).The diagnostic accuracy of magnetic resonance imaging, work perception, and social factors, in identifying symptomatic disc herniations. *Spine*, **20**(24), 2616–2625.
7. van Tulder, M.W., Assendelft, W.J., Koes, B.W. and Bouter, L.M. (1997). Spinal radiographic findings and nonspecific low back pain: a systematic review of observational studies. *Spine*, **22**(4), 427–434.
8. Luoma, K., Riihimäki, H., Luukkonen, R., Raininko, R., Viikari-Juntura, E. and Lamminen, A. (2000). Low back pain in relation to lumbar disc degeneration. *Spine*, **25**, 487–492.
9. Salminen, J.J., Erkintalo, M.O., Pentti, J., Oksanen, A. and Kormano, M.J.. (1999). Recurrent low back pain and early disc degeneration in the young. *Spine*, **24**(13), 1316–1321.
10. Boden, S.C., Davis, D.O., Dina, T.S., Patronas, N.J. and Wiesel, S.W. (1990). Abnormal magnetic-resonance scans of the lumbar spine in asymptomatic subjects. *J. Bone Joint Surg.*, **72**, 403–408.
11. Nachemson, A.L. (1992). Newest knowledge of low back pain. A critical look. *Clin. Orthop. Rel. Res.*, **279**, 8–20.
12. Boyling, J.D., Palastanga, N. and Grieve. G.P. (1994). *Grieve's Modern Manual Therapy: The Vertebral Column*. Churchill Livingstone.
13. Hides, J.A., Stokes, M.J., Saide, M., Jull, G.A. and Cooper, D.H. (1994). Evidence of multifidus wasting ipsilateral to symptoms in patients with acute low back pain. *Spine*. **19**, 165–172.
14. Hides, J.A., Richardson, C.A. and Jull, G.A.. (1996). Multifidus muscle recovery is not automatic following resolution of acute first episode low back pain. *Spine*. **21**(23), 2763–2769.

15. Gibson, J.N., Grant, I.C. and Waddell, G. (1999). The Cochrane review of surgery for lumbar disc prolapse and degenerative lumbar spondylosis. *Spine,* **24**(17), 1820–1832.
16. Clinical Standards Advisory Group report on low back pain. (1994). December, HMSO.
17. Thomas, E., Silman, A.J., Croft, P.R., Papageorgiou, A.C., Jayson, M.I. and Macfarlane, G.J. (1999). Predicting who develops chronic low back pain in primary care: a prospective study. *BMJ,* **318**(7199), 1662–1667.
18. Accident Rehabilitation and Compensation Insurance Corporation of New Zealand and the National Health Committee. (1997). *Guide to assessing psychological yellow flags in acute low back pain.* Wellington, NZ.
19. Allied Dunbar National Fitness Survey. (1992).
20. Leboeuf-Yde, C. (1999). Smoking and low back pain. A systematic literature review of 41 journal articles reporting 47 epidemiological studies. *Spine,* **24**(14), 1463–1470.
21. Scott, S.C., Goldberg, M.S., Mayo, N.E., Stock, S.R., Poitras, B. (1999). The association between cigarette smoking and back pain in adults. *Spine,* **24**(11), 1090–1098.
22. Office for National Statistics Omnibus Survey (1998)
23. WHO. (1980). *International Classification of Impairments, Disability and Handicaps.* World Health Organisation, Geneva.
24. Waddell, G. (1987). A new clinical model for the treatment of low back pain. *Spine,* **12**, 632–644.
25. Young, A. (1996). *A study to rationalise the management of acute low back pain at Kettering Hospital.* Personal correspondence.
26. Dickson, A. (1998). Routine Referral for X-ray for Patients Presenting to GPs with LBP. Oxford Spine Research Group http://www.osrg.com/index3.htm.
27. Frost, H., Lamb, S.E. and Shackleton, C. (2000). Functional restoration programme for chronic low back pain. A prospective outcome study. *Physiotherapy,* **86**(6), 285–293.
28. Burton, A.K., Waddell, G., Burtt, R. and Blair, S. (1996). Patient educational material in the management of low back pain in primary care. *Bull. Hosp. Jt Dis.,* **55**(3), 138–141. (Review).
29. Burton, A.K., Waddell, G., Tillotson, K.M. and Summerton, N. (1999). Information and advice to patients with back pain can have a positive effect. A randomized controlled trial of a novel educational booklet in primary care. *Spine,* **24**(23), 2484–2491.
30. Waddell, G., Feder, G. and Lewis, M. (1997). Systematic reviews of bed rest and advice to stay active for acute low back pain. *Br. J. Gen. Practice,* **47**, 647–652.
31. Frost, H., Klaber Moffett, J.A., Moser, J.S, and Fairbank, J.C. (1995). Randomised controlled trial for evaluation of fitness programme for patients with chronic low back pain. *BMJ.* **310**(6973),151–154.
32. Klaber-Moffett, J.A., Torgerson, D., Bell-Syer, S., Jackson, D., Llywelyn-Phillips, H., Farrin, A. and Barber, J. (1999). Randomised control trial of exercise for low back pain: clinical outcome, costs and preferences. *BMJ,* **319**, 279–283.

Chapter 4

Rehabilitation of the Chronic Pain Patient

Alison Hatfield and Richard Bartley

The most effective way to manage patients with chronic low back pain is probably to prevent their back pain becoming chronic in the first place! Judicious advice for acute back pain sufferers to remain active, avoid bed rest and with access to physiotherapy or other manual therapy for those that need it, could help to substantially reduce low back pain disability. Vigilance and early detection of signs of illness behaviour is also important, although it is accepted that prevention of chronic back pain may not be possible in every case.

The reasons why some patients go on to develop chronic low back pain, whilst others do not, are complex and the subject of much debate. It is important to recognize that many patients who are classified as chronic back sufferers do not in fact have continual back pain, rather that they experience intermittent episodes and can lead normal lives at other times.

The chronic pain patient on the other hand becomes trapped in a spiral of unremitting pain, stress, anxiety and frustration that can last months, and in many cases, years. How these patients can be best managed is still open to debate.

Rehabilitation

Rehabilitation in the form of exercise classes has recently become accepted as an effective approach to managing patients with chronic low back pain. Rehabilitation may be delivered in combination with cognitive behavioural therapy and long-term medication.

The basis for this approach lies with the fact that back pain leads to immobility, stiffness and eventually, a chronic pain cycle, where attempts by the patient to mobilize result in more pain. This cycle may persist until the patient has become unfit to work and lead a normal life.

The patient's beliefs about pain and their response to injury are important contributors to the chronic pain cycle, both in initiating and perpetuating it. Addressing these psychosocial factors, as described in the preceding chapter, can break the cycle and enable the patient to improve their levels of fitness and pain tolerance. Changes in nerve transmission

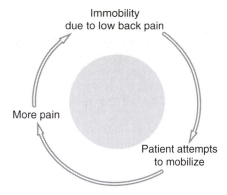

Figure 4.1 Chronic pain cycle.

may also have a role in perpetuating the pain cycle and these may be modified with medication when combined with exercise.

The responsibility for pain management needs to be handed back to the patient. The aim of rehabilitation is to improve current levels of function and reduce distress rather than to cure pain. It is important to inform the patient, before embarking on a rehabilitation programme, that improvement is often gradual with the patient likely to experience flare ups, particularly in the early stages of the programme.

The rehabilitation goals for patients with chronic low back pain are to:

1. Increase the range and level of daily activities including reducing time spent resting and lying down.
2. Increase physical fitness in terms of power, endurance and flexibility.
3. Improve management of pain by the patient:
    (a) reduce the tendency to overdo things by improved pacing activities;
    (b) learn and utilize a relaxation technique;
    (c) increase confidence in ability to function and cope.
4. Improve sleep and eliminate inappropriate sedatives.
5. Rationalize and reduce powerful analgesics, antidepressants and tranquillizers.
6. Eliminate unnecessary aids such as corsets, collars and crutches.
7. Return to work if appropriate.
8. Reduce long-term health care utilization.

Functional restoration programmes (FRPs)

These are normally managed by a physician-led team, including physiotherapists, occupational therapists and clinical psychologists. Patients are placed on a three or four week intensive exercise programme, attending daily up to five days a week.

Patients are introduced to the concepts of pain management and embark on a progressive exercise programme designed to increase their tolerance to exercise. Although physiotherapists are usually the main facilitators, cognitive behavioural therapists provide input to help deal with patient's problems and in particular to address issues of demotivation and anger. The latter being necessary due to patients often being passed along from one clinician to another without any effective management plan being instigated.

The cognitive behavioural approach places emphasis on training the patient to monitor and to deal with unhelpful beliefs and reactions to pain. The patient is assisted in developing ways of challenging and then changing these reactions to more helpful responses.[1]

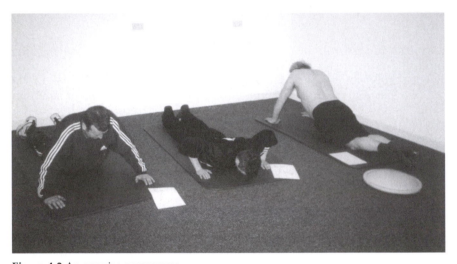

Figure 4 2 An exercise programme.

Exercise compliance decreases rapidly over time even amongst patients who know that adhering to their prescribed exercise regimen will lead to symptom relief. Motivation is particularly difficult to attain when an immediate benefit is unlikely or impossible.[2] The FRP team encourage patients to take a positive approach. For example, reinforcing that regular, paced activity is preferable to lying down for excessive periods during the day and complaining about pain.

The FRP programme should be customized to the patient's needs and the starting point will depend on the individual's abilities and personal goals. The success of exercise therapy depends on the exercises being tailored to the type and stage of the disorder, being of the proper intensity and performed with the correct techniques. They also need to be performed regularly and consistently.

Patients are encouraged to increase activities wherever possible and be advised that they are not doing further damage to their back, even if they suffer some stiffness and pain subsequently.

Compliance is also related to the patient's health beliefs. Those who believe that health depends on their own behaviour appear to be more compliant than those who think that they can do little by themselves to improve their condition and rely on their fate, institutions, medicine, or other persons. Compliance is more likely when given clear instructions and when the rationale and benefits of the prescribed regimen are understood.

Information required for planning rehabilitation for chronic back pain:

- Cause of pain: what started it (this may give any insight into patient's worries and any maintaining factors – does it date from an accident, is there ongoing litigation).
- Duration of pain, pattern of pain through the day – precipitating and relieving factors.
- Current level of activity (baseline for rehabilitation): walking distance and use of walking aids, ability to carry out personal and domestic activities of daily living.
- Sleep – is the patient woken by pain – if so chronic tiredness is likely to exacerbate the symptoms.
- Mood.
- Social situation: family, housing, finances, work satisfaction.
- Use of alcohol and drugs.
- Other medical problems, e.g. ischaemic heart disease, which may limit exercises and the use of drugs.
- Do they need to drive or operate machinery as their ability to do this safely may be affected.

Providing the goals are meaningful to the patient their achievement will also reinforce their efforts. Patients with low back pain have a fear of exercising and a supervised program may allay this fear and encourage these patients to develop increased strength and the ability to participate in normal daily activities.

Following attendance of the FRP, patients should perform aerobic exercise training 3 times per week doing 20–40 minutes per session starting with a warm up and then training at a heart rate 40–80% of the maximum heart rate (220-age). This maintenance programme needs to fit into the daily routine and not require too much extra time.

The evidence for FRPs

A number of studies have examined the efficacy of FRPs. Mayer (1985) and Hazard (1989) reported success rates of around 80 per cent.[3,4] However other studies since have questioned these results,[5,6] mainly because rates of return to work at 12 months were not as significant as Mayer's and Hazard's findings.

Williams et al. (1993) found that behavioural therapy as part of a FRP is an effective treatment with good short-term results: significant improvement on quality of life, physical performance, pain tolerance and distress; depression severity and confidence.[7] Both inpatients and outpatients made significant improvement in physical performance and psychological function and reduced medication use. Inpatients made greater gains and maintained them better.[8] They also went on to use less healthcare resources. These findings are supported in other studies.[9,10]

Frost et al. (2000)[11] undertook a longitudinal prospective study to assess the clinical benefits of a newly established FRP for patients with chronic low back pain. The overall aim of the programme was to improve function and encourage patients to take a more active role in their own management. At one year, scores for disability, psychological distress and depression showed small to moderate improvement. This study provides some support for the use of FRPs but more research is needed to satisfy purchasers and providers that they are an important tool in managing chronic low back pain.

Referral to FRP programmes

Early detection of patients with signs of chronic illness behaviour is important if disability due to low back pain is to be reduced. A number of premorbid factors are now recognized as warning signs ('yellow flags'). Yet, however well the GP is able to identify these patients, his or her ability to manage them successfully depends on the availability of specialized chronic pain programmes or services.

A number of multidisciplinary units now exist in NHS regions across the United Kingdom. These are often reconstituted pain clinics which provide a wide range of services, including FRPs, post-operative symptom control, neurostimulation (TENS, dorsal column implants) and standard analgesic regimes.[15]

Their strength lies in their multiprofessional approach with strategic planning for patients with chronic pain. Details of these units are available from the Pain Society of Great Britain and Northern Ireland, 9 Bedford Square, London WC1B 3RA.

In areas where no such facilities are available, local services could be organized to provide local FRP-type programmes. A number of primary care centres have access to clinical psychologists and physiotherapists and with adequate planning and resources their patients with chronic low back pain could be managed effectively within the community.

Using drugs to assist the rehabilitation process

Many clinicians integrate rehabilitation programmes with a long-term drug management for chronic low back pain.

NSAIDs

There is evidence that non-steroidal anti-inflammatory drugs (NSAIDs) are effective for chronic low back pain and that the different types of anti-inflammatory are equally effective. There is limited evidence that paracetamol is equally effective as Diflunisal. There is limited evidence that muscle relaxants are effective for chronic low back pain.[9]

Antidepressants

Tricyclic antidepressants have been found beneficial for chronic pain sufferers[12,13] both for those who are and those who are not depressed although there is conflicting evidence.[9] They facilitate sleep and relaxation but need to be taken regularly for several weeks. Patients should be warned about sedation, dry mouth and constipation and reassured that they are not addictive.

Combining drugs

Care should be advised when using multiple drug regimens. Drug changes should be made one at a time. Patients should be warned to observe for drowsiness and to avoid driving if affected. Tricyclic antidepressants have been shown to impair tracking ability although the effect largely resolves after a week's treatment owing to adaptation.[14]

Accidents may result from falls caused by postural hypotension mediated by the anti-alpha adrenoceptor effect of antidepressants and rarely by drug-induced cardiac arrhythmias and convulsions. Combinations of drugs with central nervous system or hypotensive side-effects should be avoided.

Summary

The management of chronic back pain should be focused on increasing the range and level of daily activities through pacing and prioritizing important activities. Pain alleviation should not be the goal, but rather it should be to encourage patients to cope better with their symptoms and to be more active. Some evidence has been found for the benefits of FRPs which combine exercise therapy with a cognitive-behavioural approach. A multiprofessional approach enables strategic planning and delivery of these programmes.

References

1. Pither, C.E., Nicholas, M.K. (1991). Psychological approaches in chronic pain management. *Br. Med. Bull.*, **47**(3), 743–761.
2. Friedrich, M., Gittler, G., Halberstadt, Y. *et al.* (1998). Combined exercise and motivation programme: effect on the compliance and level of disability of patients with chronic low back pain: a randomised controlled trial. *Arch. Phys. Med. Rehabil.*, **79**, 475–487.

3. Mayer, T.G., Gatchel, R.J., Kishino, N., Keeley, J., Capra, P., Mayer, H., Barnett, J. and Mooney, V. (1985). Objective assessment of spine function following industrial injury. A prospective study with comparison group and one-year follow-up. *Spine*, **10**(6), 482–493.

4. Hazard, R.G., Fenwick, J.W., Kalisch, S.M., Redmond, J., Reeves, V., Reid, S. and Frymoyer, J.W. (1989). Functional restoration with behavioural support. A one-year prospective study of patients with chronic low-back pain. *Spine*, **14**(2), 157–161.

5. Oland, G and Tveiten, G. (1991). A trial of modern rehabilitation for chronic low back pain and disability: vocational outcome and effect on pain modulation. *Spine*, **16**, 457–459.

6. Teasell, R.W. and Harth, M. (1996). Functional restoration. Returning patients with chronic low back pain to work – revolution or fad? *Spine*. **21**(7), 844–847. Review.

7. Williams, A.C.D.E.C., Nicholas, M.K., Richardson, P.H., et al., (1993) Evaluation of a cognitive behavioural programme for rehabilitating patients with chronic pain. *Br. J. Gen. Practice*, **43**, 513–518.

8. Williams, A.C.D.E.C., Richardson, P.H., Nicholas, M.K., et al., (1996) Inpatient vs. outpatient pain management: results of a randomised controlled trial. *Pain*, **66**, 13–22.

9. van Tulder, M.W., Koes, B.W. and Bouter, L.M. (1997). Conservative treatment of acute and chronic non-specific low back pain. A systematic review of RCTs of the most common interventions. *Spine*, **22**(18), 2128–2156.

10. Bendix, A.F., Bendix, T., Lund, C. *et al.* (1997). Comparison of three intensive programs for chronic low back pain patients: a prospective, randomized observer blinded study with one year follow up. *Scand. J. Rehab. Med.*, **29**, 81–89.

11. Frost, H., Lamb, S.E. and Shackleton, C. (2000). Functional restoration programme for chronic low back pain. A prospective outcome study. *Physiotherapy*, **86**(6), 288–293.

12. Pheasant, H., Bursk, A., Goldfarb, J. *et al.* (1983). Amitriptyline and chronic low back pain – a randomised double blind crossover study. *Spine*, **8**(5), 552–557.

13. Ward, N. (1986). Tricyclic antidepressants for chronic back pain – mechanisms of action and predictors of response. *Spine*, **11**(7), 661–665.

14. Edwards, J.G. (1995). Depression, antidepressants and accidents. *BMJ*, **311**; 887.

15. Booker, K. and Cooper, R. (1999). Management of the chronic pain patient in primary and tertiary care. In *Practical Problems*, Series three. Arthritis Research Campaign.

Section 3

Nerve Root Pain

Chapter 5

Nerve Root Compression and Cauda Equina Syndrome

Richard Bartley

Nerve root compression

Introduction

Mechanical compression of a nerve root results in sensory or motor changes, or both. It is known that simple mechanical pressure alone should not lead to the sensation of pain.[1] For pain to exist additional factors must be involved.

It appears that inflammatory mediators are probably the main cause of nerve pain.[2] Severe and sudden compression of a nerve root may cause local oedema and the release of noxious chemicals such as prostaglandins and substance P. These inflammatory agents may remain active for several weeks. Further insult to the nerve root (e.g. dragging the nerve root across a space-occupying mass when changing from sitting to standing) may cause further release of these chemicals. The dorsal root ganglion is much more pain sensitive to compression than peripheral nerves and may become involved in lateral disc protrusions.

There are also some circumstances where nerve root pain may be associated with disturbed vascularity due to arterial sclerosis and possibly because of disturbance of cerebrospinal fluid (CSF) flow outside the nerve root or fluid flow within it.

It is common in clinical practice to find by chance, patients with sequestrated disc material compressing one or more nerve roots in the vertebral canal or exit foramina without pain or disability. Conversely there are other patients who complain bitterly of unbearable leg pain in the absence of any imaging evidence of nerve root compression. This paradox means that management should be based on symptoms rather than radiological findings alone.

Clinical presentation

Nerve root pain is usually in a dermatomal distribution. That is anterior thigh (L3 and L4), shin and dorsomedial foot (L5), calf and plantar and lateral foot (S1). Sometimes S1 pain is just felt in the posterior thigh (perhaps because of sacral root involvement). The pain is severe with a funny sensation, parasthesia and numbness.

In contrast, neurogenic claudication symptoms are commonly not in a dermatomal distribution and may involve the whole of the lower limb. This may be experienced as a pain or heaviness. Even articulate patients struggle to describe this sensation. It is often accompanied by back pain and can be confused with the symptoms of osteoarthritis of the hip.

The vertebral canal cross-sectional area has considerable individual variation. Patients with wide canals can avoid nerve root compression even when there is substantial herniation, whilst those with narrow canals are much more vulnerable to symptomatic disc prolapses and neurogenic claudication.

It is common with nerve root pain for only one leg to be symptomatic. Pain extending below the gluteal crease, but not below the posterior knee crease, is rarely due to a nerve root pain. An exception to this is anterior thigh pain, which may indicate one of the following:

- an L3 root lesion (roughly 2 per cent of nerve root lesions will involve the L3/4 level of the lumbar spine);
- L4 root pain that is not severe enough to extend below the knee;
- referred pain from an osteoarthritic hip.

The former two presentations can be confirmed by performing the straight leg raise and femoral stretch tests which are described later.

Numerous pain-sensitive structures in the lumbar spine may result in referred pain into the buttock and thigh.[3] This is not the same as radiating pain due to nerve root compression. With referred pain, the low back pain symptoms will be more dominant. Focal nerve root pain is nearly always more severe than any accompanying low back or buttock pain, and is frequently present in the absence of any central low back symptoms. This is why terms such as sciatica can be misleading, the term being indiscriminately used to describe any type of leg pain.

Nerve root pain may be accompanied by a scoliosis of the spine. The scoliosis may be to the same side of the painful leg or to the opposite side. This compensatory scoliosis has been for some years explained as a reflex action to take the nerve root away from the offending mass. The ipsilateral shift indicating a disc herniation lying medial to the nerve root, a contralateral shift indicating a disc herniation lateral to the nerve root. These theories have now largely been discredited. The scoliosis may simply be due to indiscriminatory unilateral reflex hypertonicity in the spinal extensor muscles which flanks the lumbar spine.

Not all patients with nerve root pain will exhibit neurological signs. A study carried out at the Nuffield Orthopaedic Centre in 1998, demonstrated the presence of soft neurological signs (i.e. slight sensory, motor and/or reflex impairment) in 50 per cent of patients complaining of lower limb pain, but with no radiological evidence of focal nerve root compression.[4]

There is no consensus whether patients who present with recent foot drop, with or without nerve root pain, should be referred for emergency surgery. There is no evidence to support the view that emergency surgery is necessary in all these cases, cauda equina being an obvious exception. It is argued that the only criteria for surgery is whether the patient's leg pain cannot be adequately controlled with medication and rest. [There is a group of patients whose leg pain resolves once the foot drop has occurred. The chance of rapid recovery of the foot drop following emergency surgery is small]. It is advisable for the GP to contact the local surgeon to discuss admission in these cases.

Clinical features of nerve root compression

- The patient's leg pain will be worse than pain reported in the lumbosacral spine.
- There may be a compensatory scoliosis of the spine.
- Neurological signs may be present (e.g. hypo-reflexia, sensory loss, motor weakness).

Patients reporting bladder and/or bowel disturbances, saddle anaesthesia or progressive lower limb motor dysfunction should be investigated urgently for possible cauda equina syndrome (see later in this chapter).

Aetiology

The reported leg pain may develop suddenly, with or without trauma, or gradually over a period of days or weeks. Some patients report grumbling back pain a few days prior to the onset of their leg symptoms. The literature states that 90 per cent of cases of focal nerve root compression will resolve within six weeks from time of onset,[5] although in my experience this often takes up to 12 weeks.

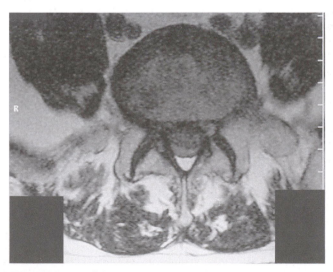

Figure 5.1 MRI axial image of disc protrusion at L4/5 causing compression of the left L5 nerve root.

The leg pain will usually be worse walking or standing and eased by lying, although some seem to be worse sitting. Some can find no relief in any position.

Leg pain worse at night, particularly if it requires the patient to wake up frequently and feel the need to walk about or sleep in a chair is a 'red flag' and should be viewed with suspicion. The intruding mass compressing the nerve root could be a primary or secondary tumour. Difficulties with micturition should be investigated for possible space-occupying lesions in the high lumbar spine, e.g. an ependymoma. Associated constitutional changes, such as unexplained sudden weight loss, extreme malaise and night sweats should also raise suspicion of a sinister pathology.

Signs of suspected serious underlying cause for leg pain (Red Flags)

- Pain at night requiring the patient to get out of bed.
- Problems with micturition.
- Associated constitutional changes, e.g. sudden unexplained weight loss, malaise.

Investigations

Imaging

The optimum investigation for a nerve root lesion is magnetic resonance imaging (MRI). It is important to obtain axial (transverse) views so that the exiting nerve roots and the lateral recesses within the spinal canal can be adequately visualized. Computerized tomography (CT) scans are sometimes used although this carries an increased radiation exposure risk. Myelography is seldom used these days. Plain X-rays have no value, other than to exclude sinister pathology or fractures (although the sensitivity of plain X-rays for sinister pathology is inferior to MRI). CT/ myelography is used in complex cases when there has been previous surgery or where MRI is contraindicated.

All radiological investigations should be used to confirm or refute clinical findings. Nerve root pain cannot be identified with imaging alone.

Clinical tests

The straight leg raise is the most reliable clinical test available.[6] It should be performed with the patient supine on an examination couch. Care should be taken not to be too vigorous in carrying out the test, particularly with patients with potentially severe root compression. It is important to test for two findings:

1. a straight leg raise of less than 45 degrees from the neutral position (i.e. the leg at 0 degrees elevation);

2. reproduction of the patients *leg* pain (i.e. not back pain) when performing the test.

The straight leg raise test (SLR) is performed in various different ways by different practitioners. It is preferable to flex the hip and knee first and then 'gently' extend the knee. If this produces pain the leg should be lowered and the procedure repeated until the leg is straight. This will then be the SLR measurement (see Fig. 5.2).

This method is useful because it allows the clinician to determine whether the patient has an osteoarthritic hip and it can help provide a more accurate reading in chronic low back pain patients who are often not familiar with this method and do not over-react as soon as a hand is placed on the heel.

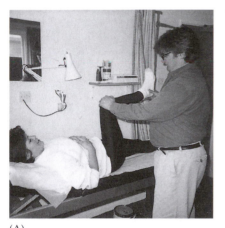 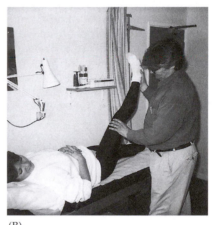

(A)   (B)

Figure 5.2 (A) First part of the straight leg raise test (flex the hip and knee). (B) Second part of the straight leg raise test (straighten the leg).

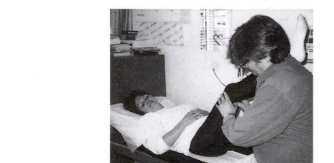

Figure 5.3 The Bowstring test.

A straight leg raise of 45 degrees or more is likely to exclude nerve root compression. Equivocal results around 45 degrees of elevation can be re-tested by flexing the knee 10 degrees during the straight leg raise test and pressing firmly with the thumbs in the posterior thigh about 2 cm above the knee crease (Bowstring test, see Fig. 5.3). Reproduction of the patient's leg pain confirms nerve root compression (due to the nerve root being tensioned).

Elevation of the good leg which reproduces the patient's pain in the affected leg, is termed a positive cross-over sign. A positive cross-over sign is nearly always pathognomic of moderate to severe nerve root compression in the lumbar spine.

The L3 root can be tested using the femoral stretch test. Place the patient prone and flex the knee of the affected leg (see Fig. 5.4). Pain reproduced in the patient's anterior thigh may suggest an L3 root lesion. A positive cross-over sign may also be present with this test.

Neurological signs may also be present (although invariably they are not). Reflexes should be tested at the knee and ankle. The knee reflex tests the L3 root and the ankle reflex tests the S1 nerve root. An intact Achilles tendon reflex either indicates that the reflexes have not been compromised or that the lesion is associated with the L5 root only.

Sensation should be tested for light touch and pinprick. Stroking each dermatome with a light cotton bud will test light touch (see Fig. 5.5). A deficit may indicate an upper motor neuron lesion. The pinprick test will test fine sensation, sometimes impaired when a peripheral nerve is compressed. A sensory loss in the anterior thigh may indicate a lesion affecting the L3 root. Sensory loss of the anterior shin may reflect an L4 lesion and the outside of the foot, an L5 lesion. Sensory loss over the heel is associated with compression of the S1 root.

Motor power can be tested using the MRC Scale (see Table 5.1). The quadriceps are supplied by the L3 nerve roots and weakness may indicate a femoral nerve lesion. The ankle/foot dorsiflexors test the L4 nerve roots, the extensor hallucis longus tests the L5 root and the ankle

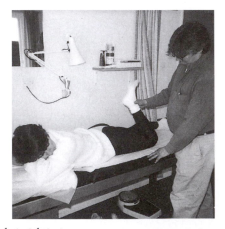

Figure 5.4 The femoral stretch test.

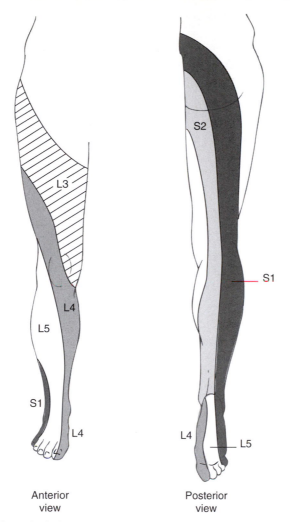

Figure 5.5 The lower limb dermatomes.

plantarflexors test the S1 root. Testing the dorsiflexors and plantarflexors in weight-bearing can be unreliable.

Lumbosacral range of movement will often be reduced in cases of focal nerve root compression. Flexion may reveal a list to the ipsilateral or contralateral side to the painful leg.

Blood tests

These should be requested if sinister underlying pathology is suspected and should include full blood count (FBC), ESR and CRP. LFTs may be requested to exclude bone disease. PSA may be considered in males over 55.

Table 5.1 The MRC scale for testing motor power

P5	Full power – able to resist
P4	Able to sustain moderate resistance
P3	Able to move the joint though its full range against gravity but cannot sustain moderate resistance
P2	Can move through full range of movement with gravity eliminated but not against gravity
P1	Visible contraction
P0	No contraction

Management

Ninety per cent of cases involving nerve root compression will resolve with time. Adequate reassurance and the judicious use of medication will usually suffice. The patient may need to take a few weeks off work but prolonged bed-rest should be discouraged (mainly to avoid the risk of deep-vein thrombosis). Adequate analgesia taken on a regular basis should suffice in most cases, reserving the opiates for those with severe pain.

The use of manipulation for these patients is not supported by current evidence and is considered to be contraindicated in patients with any neurological deficit. Traditional physiotherapy involving heat, massage and traction, may help provide some additional pain relief.

Surgery is indicated if the patient's pain cannot be adequately controlled with medication and cessation of normal activities. Surgical decompression has a typical success rate of 95 per cent. Spinal epidural carries only a 30 per cent success rate, but is less invasive. It is sometimes used as a stop-gap for patients awaiting surgery, particularly in those patients with root symptoms but no radiological signs of compression.

Other procedures include chemonucleolysis. This involves a percutaneous injection of chymopapain carried out under fluoroscopy control. The success rate is typically 75 per cent with a 1 per cent risk of discitis following the procedure. There is an even smaller risk of anaphylactic shock, which is addressed by the attendance of an anaesthetist during the procedure. Chemonucleolysis cannot be performed if the offending disc hernia has sequestrated, in other words the hernia must be contained (see Table 5.2).

Table 5.2 Management of leg pain secondary to nerve root compression

Rest and adequate medication to control the pain	90% success rate
Physiotherapy/chiropractic/osteopathy	success rate not known
Surgical decompression	95% success rate
Chemical lysis	75% success rate
Epidural	30% success rate

Four types of lumbar disc herniation

Normal disc

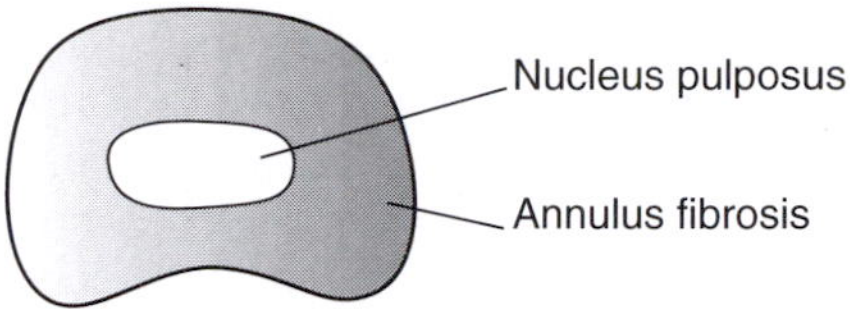

Nucleus pulposus

Annulus fibrosis

**Diffuse bulge
(disc distension)**

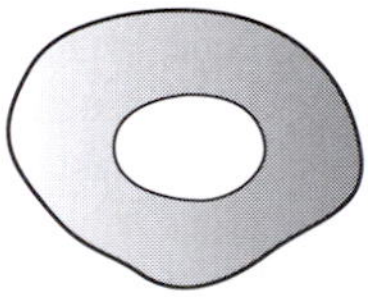

Related to natural ageing – a common finding in the asymptomatic population

Prolapse

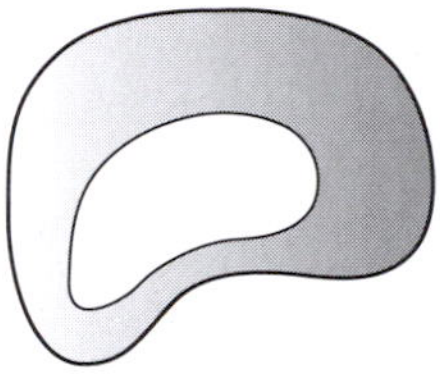

An extrusion of nucleus pulposus without breach of the outer annulus pulposus, causing the annulus to buckle in a central-posterior, a posterio-lateral or far lateral direction

Contained extrusion

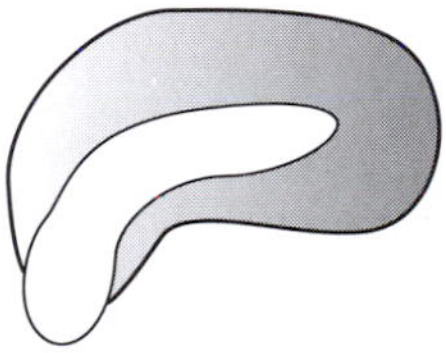

Extrusion of nucleus pulposus via a breach through the annulus fibrosis, with the nucleus pulposus remaining in contact with the main body of the disc

Non-contained extrusion (sequestration)

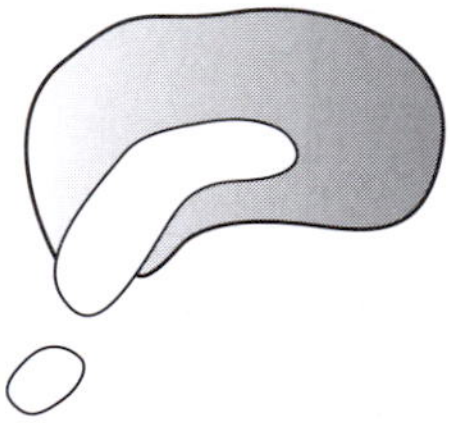

Extrusion of nucleus pulposus which separates from the main body of the disc

Figure 5.6 Four types of lumbar disc herniation.

Recovery from surgery usually takes two to three months or longer. Recovery from percutaneous chemonucleolysis can take up to one week. Reoccurrence of the clinical problem is not common with either procedure. Physical therapy may be necessary for some post-operative patients who develop scarring around the nerve root. These usually present six weeks post-operatively with a limited straight leg raise.

Reoccurrence of nerve root compression is not common. However some individuals do go on to experience one or more episodes following an initial episode of neuralgic leg pain. Ultimately this may lead the surgeon to consider performing a spinal fusion, with a typical success rates of around 65 per cent. Alternatively the patient may embark on intensive physiotherapy rehabilitation, aimed at restoring spinal range of movement, adequate straight leg raises and, most importantly, developing the spinal extensor and trunk musculature to give the patient's spine greater stability.

Cauda equina syndrome

This syndrome is a surgical emergency. It is the acute compression of the spinal nerves in the lower part of the spinal canal, most commonly caused by a large central disc prolapse, but can arise from other pathology such as spinal stenosis, infection, tumour or trauma. It is almost always characterized by the following:

- bilateral leg pain (patients reporting bilateral leg pain should always raise a 'red flag' for cauda equina syndrome);
- bladder and bowel disturbance;
- saddle anaesthesia;

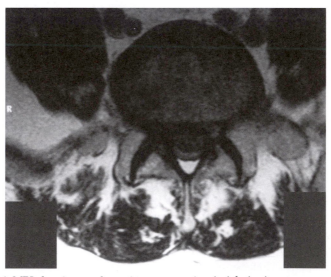

Figure 5.7 A MRI showing cauda equina compression (axial view).

- at least pericoccygeal sensory loss and in many cases, perianal numbness;
- varying degrees of loss of lower extremity motor or sensory function.

It is important to note that there may be little or no back pain. Permanent damage to the bladder can occur within twelve hours of onset unless surgery is performed.[7,8]

Presentation

The spinal cord ends at about L1/2. It then forms a 'horse's tail' (*cauda equina*) of descending nerve roots that exit the spine via the lumbar intervertebral foramen between each vertebra, the angle of these descending roots becoming more acute from above downwards. This leash of nerve endings are surrounded by the dural-arachnoid sheath and this constitutes the cauda equina.

Sudden compression of the cauda equina by a central lumbar disc prolapse can lead to the following symptoms:

- urinary retention;
- saddle anaesthesia;
- reduced rectal tone and sensory sensitivity;
- progressive sensory or motor changes in the lower limbs.

Urinary disturbances

Patients with acute low back pain may experience retention, urinary frequency, urgency and a reduced flow. These symptoms may be associated with anxiety or pain. Perner *et al.* (1997) studied the prevalence, nature and severity of lower urinary tract symptoms in 108 cases of lumbar nerve root compression without cauda equina compression.[9] Over half reported lower urinary tract symptoms, including urinary frequency, poor flow and even retention.

It is therefore important to distinguish such cases from those with neurogenic bladder disturbance due to cauda equina syndrome. It is useful to ask two questions. Firstly, does the patient have a normal feeling of a full bladder? If the response is negative, the patient should be asked whether they can feel urine passing down the urethra when they pass water. If they have cauda equina syndrome they will not have that feeling or they will not know when they have finished (or as one patient commented "I only knew when I finished when the noise stopped").

Other important indicators of possible cauda equina syndrome are:

- an extended bladder, confirmed with careful palpation of the lower abdomen;
- patient reporting an inability to pass urine for more than eight hours.

Catheterization is important to prevent permanent damage to the bladder. A residual volume of more than 150 ml of urine with catheterization would be a strong indicator of urinary retention due to cauda equina syndrome.

Bowel disturbance

Loss of anal tone and sensation can be confirmed by PR. A useful question to ask the patient is whether they can tell the difference between flatus and faeces. Failure to distinguish the two sensations in patients with severe low back pain may indicate a cauda equina syndrome.

Saddle anaesthesia

Numbness of the perineum, genitalia or anus.

Lower limb dysfunction

Patients with low back pain reporting progressive limb weakness or loss of normal sensation should be assessed thoroughly. Reflexes, sensory and motor tests should be carried out (test hip flexion, knee extension and foot dorsiflexion against resistance). The prognosis in cauda equina syndrome is worse for bladder and bowel function than for sensory or motor function.[10]

Incidence

It has been reported that one case will present annually for every 50 000 patients seen in primary care (one case for every five GP practices with a list size of 10 000 patients).[10]

Management of cauda equina syndrome

If in doubt – refer for emergency opinion! Despite Perner et al's study findings, these cases should always be thoroughly investigated.

The optimum investigation of choice is MRI. Confirmation of a large central disc prolapse compressing the cauda equina will lead to urgent discectomy either by wide laminotomy or laminectomy which is the most prudent surgical approach for this condition.[11]

Summary

- Ninety per cent of cases of nerve root pain resolve within 12 weeks from time of initial onset.
- Nerve root pain is always usually worse than any accompanying low back pain.
- The straight leg raise test (SLR) is a good indicator of a nerve root lesion.
- Reflexes, motor and sensory signs are not so reliable.
- There is no strong evidence to support the need for urgent referral for cases of foot drop for emergency surgery.
- *Cases involving bilateral leg pain, with bladder or bowel disturbance need urgent referral for a specialist opinion.*

References

1. Garfin, S.R., Rydevik, B.L. and Brown, R.A. (1988). Compressive neuropathy of spinal nerve roots: a mechanical or biological problem? *Spine*, **16**, 162–166.
2. Marshall, L.L., Trethewie, E.R. and Curtain, C.C. (1977). Chemical radiculitis. *Clin. Orthop. Rel. Res.*, **129**, 61–67.
3. McNab, I. (1977). *Backache*. Williams & Wilkins.
4. Bartley, R., Marshall, T., McNally, E., Fairbank, J.C.T. and Pynsent, P.B. (2000). Sciatica due to lumbar disc herniation. Does the degree of spinal nerve root compression correspond to symptoms, signs and disability? (in press).
5. van Tulder, M.W., Koes, B.W. and Bouter, L.M. (1996). *Low Back Pain in Primary Care: Effectiveness of Diagnostic and Therapeutic Interventions*. CIP-Gegevens Koninklijke Bibliotheeek.
6. Edgar, M.A. and Park, W.M. (1974). Induced patterns on passive straight leg raising in lower lumbar disc protrusion: a clinical, myelographic and operative study on fifty patients. *J. Bone Joint Surg.[Br]*, **56**, 658–667.
7. Cailliet, R. (1988). *Low Back Pain Syndrome*. FA Davies & Company.
8. Kennedy, J.G., Soffe, K.E., McGrath, A., Stephens, M.M., Walsh, M.G. and McManus, F. (1999). Predictors of outcome in cauda equina syndrome. *Eur. Spine J.*, **8**(4), 317–322
9. Perner, A., Andersen, J.T. and Juhler, M. (1997). Lower urinary tract symptoms in lumbar root compression syndromes. *Spine*, **22**, 2693–2697.
10. ONS. (1995). *Morbidity Statistics from General Practice, 4th National Study, 1991–1992*, Series MB5 No. 3, HMSO.
11. Esses, S. (1995). *Textbook of Spinal Disorders*. JB Lippincott.

Chapter 6

Neurogenic Claudication and Spinal Stenosis

Sunny Deo

Introduction

Spinal stenosis is a common problem which affects middle-aged and elderly patients. It may be difficult to diagnose, as a number of other conditions, such as tumours, infection and other neurological conditions, may present with similar symptoms. It is however amenable to treatment.

The subject of neurogenic claudication and its prime cause, spinal stenosis, continues to be a complex and poorly understood problem amongst those who deal with low back problems, particularly in terms of defining underlying pathology and the optimum modes of treatment.

Consensus does exist with regard to breaking down the problem into a number of subgroups and tailoring appropriate investigations and treatment depending on the subgroup of stenosis.

The terms neurogenic claudication was first coined in 1911 and that of spinal stenosis (from congenital causes) only in 1954. Developments in imaging, particularly MRI have greatly improved understanding and rationalized treatments over the last two decades.

In order to minimize confusion listed below are a number of definitions of key terms:

Spinal stenosis

This is encroachment of spinal structure (bone, joint and ligamentous) around nerve roots, the spinal cord, or in the low back, the cauda equina. The term should in theory describe the morphology of the spine as seen definitively on investigation, though it is commonly used to describe a classic pattern of symptoms and signs (see Table 6.1).

Stenosis is defined by:

1. Location
   a. cervical or lumbar spine.
   b. Specific level (s) involved e.g. L3–4.
   c. Number of levels; single or multi-level disease.
   d. Central or lateral stenosis (see below).

2. Cause   The causative classification was described by Arnoldi *et al.*[1] (see pathophysiology and Table 6.2).
3. Symptoms   Given the high proportion of patients with incidental asymptomatic stenosis (up to 40 per cent in some series) the severity of symptoms should be noted and correlated with imaging studies.

Central stenosis

Describes encroachment predominantly around the spinal canal, and can thus cause constriction around nerve roots or the whole cauda equina.

Lateral stenosis

Denotes encroachment around structures lateral to the spinal canal as nerve roots exit through the intervertebral (also termed the exit or neural) foramen. Lateral stenosis is further divided into lateral recess stenosis (between the superomedial edge of the facet joint and the back of the vertebral body or disc) and foraminal stenosis, commonly caused by an intraforaminal disc protrusion. Lateral recess stenosis is by far the commoner of the two types.

Mixed stenosis

Of both central and lateral stenosis occurs most frequently in middle-aged patients, in whom the prevalence of symptomatic stenosis is probably highest.

Tandem spinal stenosis

This is combined cervical and lumbar stenosis which in one study was found to occur in 19 per cent of patients. This will give mixed upper and lower limb features and mixed features of myelopathy and radiculopathy.

Neurogenic claudication

Describes the symptoms of a patient with lumbar spinal stenosis. Because of the lack of accurate imaging at the time when these symptoms were being attributed to spinal causes the symptom complex is somewhat

Table 6.1 Classical features of neurogenic claudication

- Back pain with radiation down the leg below the knee on walking.
- Associated neurological symptoms on walking.
- Pain relieved by sitting, bending or squatting rather than just stopping.
- No affect on walking uphill.
- Ability to cycle without symptoms.
- Lying flat may increase symptoms.
- Unlike discogenic pain bending or lifting won't worsen symptoms.

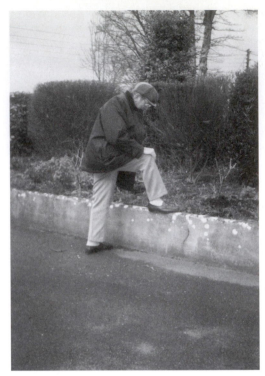

Figure 6.1 Man relieving symptoms of neurogenic claudication by resting leg on wall and flexing spine.

blurred, though there are classic features as shown in Table 6.1. Further details of symptoms are described in the symptoms section.

Pathophysiology

Depends on the mechanism and its cause.

Mechanism

The exact mechanisms for the cause of symptoms, in common with other causes of low back pain, are not fully understood and differ slightly in terms of cause. The final common factor is encroachment of spinal structures, usually abnormal, around the nerves or cauda equina. There is debate as to the cause of pain from nerve roots and the spinal structures but it is likely to be a combination of direct compression and vascular insufficiency of the nerves themselves. Primary nerve compression will cause complex, secondary changes within the nerve. The causes of nerve pain are summarized in Table 6.2.

Table 6.2 Causes of nerve pain

- Direct nerve compression.
- Nerve irritation e.g. chemical or from local inflammation.
- Compression of blood supply or venous drainage to nerves.
- Traction of the nerve.
- Primary or secondary neuritis.
- Combinations (or all) of the above.

Cause

By far the commonest cause is degenerative spinal stenosis, which can be subdivided. A comprehensive classification of common causes was published by Arnoldi *et al.*[1] and its modified version is shown in Table 6.3.

Epidemiology and natural history

The prevalence of spinal stenosis is difficult to establish, as is common with many other common conditions there are no population-based studies on which to base such information. However with increasing awareness and demands of the population and primary care workers, the incidence of diagnoses is likely to increase.

Table 6.3 Classification of spinal stenosis by cause

Congenital – Developmental stenosis	
Idiopathic	
Achondroplasia, other forms of dwarfism	
Down's syndrome, other causes of C1–2 instability	
Scoliosis	
Spondylolisthesis	
Spinal dysraphism	
Acquired stenosis	
Degenerative	Primary/Spondylosis
	Disc degeneration
	Spondylolisthesis/Scoliosis
Post-surgical	
Post-traumatic (late)	
Metabolic/endocrine	Osteoporosis
	Paget's disease
	Acromegaly
Pathologic	Rheumatoid
	Ankylosing spondylitis
	Scheurmann's disease
	Diffuse idiopathic skeletal hyperostosis
	Neoplastic (secondary tumours commonest)
	Infection – osteomyelitis, epidural abcess

In terms of degenerative stenosis, which is the commonest type, the average age of presentation is around the age of 60 with a roughly equal male to female ratio, with a slightly male bias in younger age groups. Some studies have a very significant male preponderance, however this is probably due to a skewed population e.g. studies in mining towns. Only patients who have worked in very heavy manual work are at significant (i.e. greater than 30 per cent chance) risk of developing symptomatic spinal stenosis. The proportion of patients who have had previous surgery is 15 per cent.

The natural history differs with age groups, and in general are more rapid in the younger (40–60 year) age group than older. Symptoms progress over a period of months rather than weeks and may go on for years. Johsson *et al.*[2] followed up a small population of patients with symptomatic spinal stenosis over a mean period of 4 years: 70 per cent were unchanged, 15 per cent improved and 15 per cent deteriorated. There were no dramatic deteriorations.

Clinical features

The classical symptom complex is described in Table 6.1. A significant proportion present with non-specific back and leg symptoms, and objective neurological deficits may be absent or minimal. A number of studies have tried to quantify the incidence of symptoms and signs. Another problem, as shown in Table 6.3 is that other pathologies may cause stenosis and thus these combined pathologies will alter and mix clinical features.

Symptoms

Non-specific back and leg pain have been cited as the most commonly occurring symptoms, occuring in 85–90% of patients with spinal stenosis in several studies, including a major meta-analysis.[1] Classical neurogenic claudication only occurred in 62 per cent of patients.

Objective clinical signs

Only about half of patients will have positive clinical findings in those with significant clinical symptoms and imaging evidence. Absent or reduced reflexes occur in 58 per cent, but objective myotomal weakness or dermatomal sensory disturbance occur in 40–44% and some will have

Table 6.4 Unusual presenting symptoms

- Non-specific weakness
- Dead leg
- Giving way of leg(s)
- Unsteadiness of gait
- Stiffness of legs
- Impotence
- Bladder and bowel dysfunction (sensory and motor) – 15%

Table 6.5 Objective signs of spinal stenosis

LOOK	Flexed spinal posture (may have fixed flexion at hips) 'Simian posture' Leg muscle wasting
MOVE	Reduced spinal movement especially extension Sometimes reduced straight leg raise
NEUROLOGY	Tone, including anal tone Myotomal power Dermatomal sensation including perianal sensation Reflexes

a positive straight leg raise although it is common to obtain full straight leg raises.

Clinical examination is therefore not as diagnostically important as for a disc prolapse, however it is still important in terms of differentiating between pathologies, assessing progress and changes over time. The main positive clinical features are summarized in Table 6.5.

Investigations

Magnetic resonance imaging (MRI) scanning has superseded other imaging modalities because of its ability to visualize the cauda equina and nerve roots and their relation to soft tissue and bony structures impinging on neural structures, both in the horizontal and axial planes. Other modalities still play a role, particularly in patients with absolute and relative contraindications to MRI, areas where MRI is unavailable and patients with non-titanium spinal implants *in situ*.

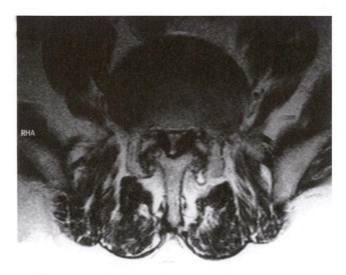

Figure 6.2 MRI of stenotic spine at the L5/S1 level (axial view).

Table 6.6 Investigations in spinal stenosis

MRI (magnetic resonance imaging)	Investigation of choice
CT (computerized tomography)	High sensitivity and low specificity
CT myelography	Probably 2nd choice
Myelography	
Plain radiography	
Electrophysiological studies	Poor sensitivity and specificity

One of the problems of imaging studies is the presence of significant stenotic changes seen on imaging studies in the normal asymptomatic population, in up to 50 per cent of over 40 year olds. Therefore the clinical features are key in determining the significance of any imaging study.

Differential diagnosis and 'red flags'

This may prove problematic as degenerative conditions of spinal structures individually, pathological conditions of the spine and conditions of the lower limbs may cause symptoms attributable to spinal stenosis. In the case of spinal conditions, stenosis and neurogenic claudication may occur secondary to other pathologies.

The variation in key symptoms and signs is summarized in Table 6.8.

Table 6.7 Common differentials of spinal stenosis

- Discogenic/lumbar spinal instability low back pain
- Prolapsed intervertebral disc
- Vascular claudication
- Hip osteoarthritis

Table 6.8 Differential diagnoses of degenerative lumbar spinal stenosis (DLSS)

Feature	DLSS	Simple	PID back pain	VASC	HIP
Predominant pain	Leg	Back	Leg	Leg	Groin/leg
Pain distribution	Post.r leg +/- foot	Back, buttock, thigh	Thigh, calf, foot	Calf +/- foot	Ant.r thigh
Onset	Months/ years	Months (episodic)	Weeks	Months	Months/ years
Tension sign (SLR)	<50%	No	>90%	No	No
Neurology	Post exercise	No	Variable	No	No
Standing/walking	Worse	Variable	Variable	Walking only	Worse

Red flag symptoms

Occasionally significant pathology will present with symptoms of neurogenic claudication or the less specific features of spinal stenosis as discussed above. The main diagnoses of note are:

Tumour – most commonly secondary of bone, though they can be primary or intradural.

Infection – usually arises as an osteomyelitis which may cause oedema or local abscess.

Pathological spine processes – Paget's of the spine, ankylosing spondylitis, post-traumatic instability.

Delay in diagnosis of tumour and infective problems is a potential catastrophe which is distressing to both patient and practitioner. It is fortunately rare and there are often clues in the past history which guide the physician e.g. past history of neoplasia or immunocompromise. Certain symptoms are deemed 'red flag' symptoms which should alert the primary care doctor to a more detailed clinical assessment and suggest the need for further urgent investigation and/or referral. In patients with low back problems these symptoms and signs are shown in Table 6.9.

Table 6.9 'Red flag' symptoms and signs in patients with low back pain

Nature of pain	Usually intense low back
	Unremitting
	Night pain
	Onset: over days and weeks vs weeks or months
	No previous history of back problems/trauma/strain
Neurological deficit	Unrelenting and progressive neurological deficits
	Leg symptoms progressing to bowel and bladder symptoms
	No relation to activity
	Bilateral symptoms
	Complete inability to walk due to weakness (not pain)
Associated symptoms	Usually NOT a feature of spinal stenosis
	Constitutional upset, fever, weight loss, anorexia

A potential diagnosis of tumour or infection should trigger a thorough clinical evaluation, urgent blood, urine and imaging investigations and appropriate referral as necessary.

Treatment options and their results

Treatment options can be broadly divided into non-operative and operative and are summarized in Table 6.10. Unfortunately because of the variety of sub-groups, anatomic locations (single or multiple levels,

Table 6.10 Treatment modalities in lumbar spinal stenosis

Non-operative	Operative
Activity modification	Lumbar decompression (LD)
Simple analgesia	LD with discectomy
Non-steroidal anti-inflammatory drugs	LD with spinal fusion
Physiotherapy	
Chiropractic/osteopathy	lumbar decompression options:
Functional restoration programme	(1) limited vs wide decompression
Epidural injection	(2) single vs multiple level LD
Calcitonin	(3) central vs lateral vs combined LD

central versus lateral compression) many smaller studies do not provide useful evidence for particular treatment modalities as the entry criteria are too heterogeneous. Interpretation of evidence, particularly for non-operative treatments, especially combinations of treatment, is sparse if not absent. There have been larger studies on the results of operative management and some important meta-analyses.

The most common combination of treatment in the UK currently is the first 4 modalities in the non-operative section. The role of chiropractic and osteopathy specifically for lumbar spinal stenosis hasn't been evaluated. For 'mild' disease these treatments have a good track record and results at one year with about 70–80% noting a significant improvement. This was not so in patients with more significant presenting symptoms and signs.[3]

Epidural injection has been widely used and overall is thought to give significant long-term improvement in 20–30% and temporary improvement, of less than 3 months, in a similar proportion.

Calcitonin was used initially in Pagetic stenosis with dramatic effect, but its wider use has not been validated to date, with good or excellent results in only 30–50% at best.

Combinations of these treatments have produced better results in individual units but have not been reproduced.

From major meta-analyses of operative treatment the results of spinal stenosis seem somewhat disappointing, with a drop in the rates of good and excellent outcome in the 1990s compared to the perhaps more optimistic results of the 1970s and 1980s, probably in part to better subjective scoring systems. The general consensus is that 65–75% of patients will have a good or excellent medium and long term outcome.[3,4,5] Significant surgical morbidity occurs in 10–15% of patients and the risk increases with age, stenosis severity and co-morbidity. Leg and claudicating symptoms do best with surgery. Only 50–60% of patients have significant improvement of back pain and 33% will have significant low back pain at one year post-op. Both patient and operation selection are key factors in optimizing results. There is no evidence backing the routine use of either wide laminectomy or spinal fusion procedures, though these are certainly used in individual cases as indicated.

Indications for investigation and referral to a spine surgeon

In general the indications for investigation (i.e. MRI scan) are:

- Severe symptoms, particularly neurologic symptoms, which may require surgery.
- Symptoms and signs which are worrying – the red flag is waving (see above).
- Symptoms and signs progressing despite non-operative treatments. A trial of 3 months, depending on symptom severity is worthwhile.

Indications for surgery are similar. There is no firm indication for surgery based on severity of pain or neurogenic claudication distance; these are individually based factors. Significant and worsening neurological function is a very strong indicator for a decompression.

Summary

- Lumbar spinal stenosis is common – the majority of people with stenosis are probably minimally or non-symptomatic.
- Patients report pain in the legs on walking which is relieved by flexion (e.g. sitting down or leaning on a wall or supermarket trolley).
- Symptoms may be confused with or caused by a number of spinal or extra-spinal problems.
- Symptomatic stenosis has a number of causes and sub-types which are clinically difficult to determine. There is a spectrum of disease severity. It is difficult to predict progression (or regression).
- Aims of management are:
  - diagnose and exclude spine tumour/infection/cord compression;
  - arrange investigations as necessary;
  - commence non-operative treatments; refer to a spine surgeon if symptoms are significant and progressing.

References

1. Arnoldi, C.C., Brodsky, A.E., Cauchoix, J. *et al.* (1976). Lumbar spine stenosis and nerve root entrapment syndromes. Definitions and classification. *Clin. Orthop.*, **115**, 4–5.
2. Johsson, K., Rosen, I., Volen, A. (1993). The natural course of lumbar spinal stenosis. *Acta Orthop. Scand. Suppl.*, **251**, 67–68.
3. Atlas, S.J., Deyo, R.A., Keller, R.B. *et al.* (2000). Surgical and non-surgical management of lumbar spine stenosis: four years from the marine lumbar spine study. *Spine*, **25**(5), 556–562.
4. Turner, J.A., Ersek, M., Herron, L. and Deyo, R.A. (1992). Surgery for spinal stenosis. *Spine*, **17**(1), 1–7.
5. Katz, J.N., Lipson, S.J., Chang, L.C., Levine, S.A., Fossel, A.H. and Liang, M.H. (1996). Seven to 10-year outcome of decompressive surgery for degenerative lumbar spinal stenosis. *Spine*, **21**(1), 92–97.

Suspected Serious Pathology

Chapter 7

Inflammatory Causes of Low Back Pain

Sally Edmonds

Introduction

The distinction between mechanical and inflammatory causes of back pain is often difficult to make on clinical grounds alone, and given that investigations in both conditions are likely to be normal, particularly early on in the course of the disease, the diagnosis of the inflammatory disorders is frequently delayed, sometimes by years. This can have significant implications especially for young patients, and it is therefore important to have a high index of suspicion and to be aware of pointers that would direct the clinician towards a diagnosis of inflammatory, rather than simple mechanical back pain.

The inflammatory group of diseases that can cause back pain are known as the 'spondyloarthropathies',[1] and include ankylosing spondylitis (AS), reactive arthritis (ReA), enteropathic arthritis (arthritis associated with inflammatory bowel disease), psoriatic arthritis (PsA) and undifferentiated spondyloarthropathy, a subgroup that has only recently been recognized.[2] All of these conditions are associated with sacroiliitis, which in AS is almost always bilateral but in the other conditions is often unilateral. The spondyloarthropathies also have other clinical features in common, such as peripheral oligoarthritis predominantly of the lower extremities, enthesopathy (inflammation of where tendon or ligament attaches to bone), anterior uveitis and a striking association with HLA-B27. Amongst the white population, the spondyloarthropathies are amongst the commonest of the rheumatic diseases with a calculated prevalence of 1.9 per cent.[3]

Reports have suggested that a GP is likely to see two patients with known AS each year[4] and one new case approximately every 5–10 years.[5] Although the diagnosis of inflammatory back pain may be delayed, it is unlikely that many cases are being overlooked in general practice.[6] In Colin's study in 1977, 313 back pain sufferers completed a screening questionnaire for inflammatory back pain.[7] This was positive in 46 patients (15 per cent) who were invited for further examination. Only two of these had definite AS. Eighteen (39 per cent) of these 46 had other features associated with a spondyloarthropathy. The authors suggest that up to 5 per cent of back pain sufferers may have a mild form of AS that may never progress to ankylosis, but for whom treatment as if they had AS may be of benefit. It is therefore important to try and identify this group of patients.

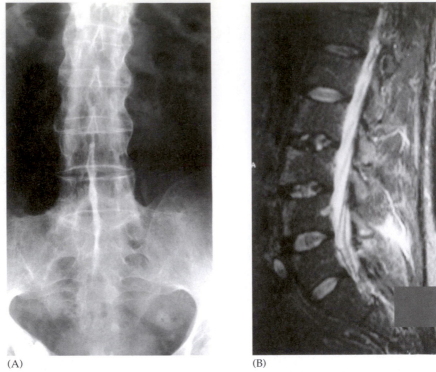

(A)   (B)

Figure 7.1 (A and B) Plain X-ray and MRI of spine with ankylosing spondylitis (the latter showing Romanus lesions in the vertebral bodies, a sign of inflammatory disease).

Making the diagnosis

The history

There are a number of features that, if present in the clinical history, should alert one to the possibility of an inflammatory cause for the patients' back pain.

Firstly, if the onset of the back pain was before the age of 40, an inflammatory cause should be considered. Children or teenagers with a spondyloarthropathy or 'enthesitis-related' arthritis are more likely to present with a peripheral arthritis or an enthesitis than low back pain, but may subsequently develop sacroiliitis.

The pain in inflammatory disorders is usually of insidious onset but may be triggered by some sort of trauma which may fool both doctor and patient into thinking that the underlying cause is a mechanical one. Pain that persists for longer than 3 months is more likely to be inflammatory, although clearly there are plenty of cases of simple back pain that have a longer history than this, and this has to be taken in context with the other clinical features.

Morning back stiffness is also a feature of inflammatory back disorders, as is improvement with exercise. I usually ask: "generally speaking, are your symptoms better if you exercise or if you rest?" Patients with simple back pain are often more comfortable resting, although this is not always a reliable sign.

If these five features of the clinical history are present, i.e. back pain that is insidious in onset, in a patient younger than 40 years, persisting for at least three months, associated with morning stiffness and improving with exercise, the diagnosis of AS is likely.[7] They have been shown to be 95 per cent sensitive and 85 per cent specific – in other words, they will only fail to detect 5 per cent of cases but make the diagnosis erroneously in 15. This is illustrated by the study quoted above,[6] where the number of 'false positives' was high.

The site of pain is not particularly helpful in differentiating mechanical from inflammatory back pain, but the latter is usually felt deep in the gluteal or sacroiliac region. Unfortunately it may also be made worse by such things as coughing or sneezing, which can further confuse.

Given the strong association, particularly in AS, with HLA-B27, it is also important to take a careful family history, asking specifically whether any other family members have had back problems from a young age, or whether there is any family history of psoriasis or inflammatory bowel disease. In addition, the patient should be asked whether they themselves have had any other features of a spondyloarthropathy, such as a swollen peripheral joint, painful red eye(s), psoriasis or diarrhoea.

What are the important features of the clinical history when making a diagnosis of inflammatory back pain?

- Was the pain of insidious onset?
- Did the pain come on before the age of 40?
- Has the pain lasted for longer than 3 months?
- Is the pain associated with significant morning stiffness?
- Does the pain get better with exercise?

The examination

The basic features of the examination of a patient with inflammatory back pain are a stiff lumbar spine, perhaps with pain on stressing the sacro-iliac joints, without any neurological deficit. Loss of movement in the lumbar spine should be assessed by checking forward flexion, lateral flexion and hyperextension – the ability of the patient to touch his toes with his knees straight should not be relied on as an indicator of good spinal mobility since a good range of movement in the hips can compensate for loss of movement in the lumbar spine and vice versa. Instead, the 'modified' Schober's test is quite useful: with the patient standing erect, mark the skin overlying the fifth lumbar vertebra (usually at the level of the posterior superior iliac spine or 'dimples of Venus') and place another mark 10 cm above this in the midline.

Ask the patient to bend forwards as far as they can without bending their knees and measure the new distance between the two marks. In health, the distance should increase by some 50–100%, i.e. to between

15 and 20 cm – anything less than this suggests active inflammatory disease (it is helpful to repeat the test two or three times as patients with mechanical back pain improve slightly when they are warmed up). A more formal approach to assessing mobility in AS has now been validated – the Bath Ankylosing Spondylitis Radiology Index,[8] but is too lengthy to be useful in the GP's surgery where the modified Schober's test should suffice.

The sacroiliac joints are very difficult to assess clinically, partly because they have minimal movement. Localized tenderness over the sacroiliac joints may be present but really doesn't provide the examiner with much useful information. Pain may be induced by trying to compress the pelvis or by distracting it and pushing it across the iliac blades. Flexing the hip and knee and forcibly adducting the leg across to the contralateral iliac fossa causes similar distraction of the pelvis and may also induce pain. However, these tests are rather non-specific and are, I think, of limited value in the clinic.

Other clinical features that may be associated with a spondyloarthropathy should be actively sought during the physical examination. These include swollen peripheral joint(s), enthesopathy, rash, nail changes and red eyes (I have had patients in my clinic who have ignored a red eye!). In particular, psoriasis of the scalp, umbilicus or natal cleft is often ignored or missed.

What is the most useful examination technique that can be done in the surgery?

- The simplest and quickest way of assessing pure lumbar spine movement is to do the modified Schober's test.

Investigations

It is, of course, possible to diagnose a spondyloarthropathy without any evidence of inflammation in the back. Although sacroiliitis is pathognomonic of AS,[9] patients with any of the other spondyloarthropathies may never develop any sacro-iliac joint inflammation. However, if one is talking about inflammatory back pain *per se*, the diagnosis of this rests upon radiological evidence of sacroiliitis – either unilateral or bilateral. In AS, sacroiliitis is usually bilateral.[10]

The plain radiograph is often of limited use in identifying sacroiliitis in the early stages of the disease, before bony changes have occurred, although in practice this is still frequently done. It can take up to 8 years for bony changes to become evident on plain X-ray. Magnetic resonance imaging (MRI) is able to pick up early inflammatory changes in the sacroiliac joints and we are using this now almost routinely. Squaring of the vertebrae on the lateral radiograph may be seen relatively early in the course of inflammatory back disease, particularly in AS. Syndesmophytes are also a specific feature of AS, but are not part of the diagnostic criteria, because their often late onset precludes early diagnosis. A good review of the radiological diagnosis of the spondyloarthropathies has recently been written.[11]

Blood tests are more often than not of little use in making the diagnosis of inflammatory back pain, and the blood count, ESR and CRP are usually normal. The thorny question of whether or not it is useful to know the patients' HLA-B27 status then arises. In a patient whose clinical picture fits with a diagnosis of inflammatory back pain, and who has radiological evidence of sacroiliitis, there is little additional useful information to be derived from knowing their HLA typing.

The indiscriminate typing of patients with musculoskeletal complaints is not warranted either, given the fact that HLA-B27 occurs in one of every 13–14 healthy individuals, and that the overwhelming majority (98–99%) of HLA-B27-positive individuals do not have a spondylo-arthropathy.[12] However, HLA-B27 typing can provide diagnostic infor-mation in certain circumstances. For example, when a family member of a patient with AS has symptoms of inflammatory spinal disease and there is no radiological evidence of sacroiliitis, or in a young patient with oligoarthritis accompanied by inflammatory eye disease. In other words, when the clinical suspicion is high, but a firm diagnosis has not been made by other means, HLA-B27-positivity would lend support to the diagnosis of inflammatory back disease.

Which investigations should the GP organize?

- Probably none. If the clinical history and examination are suggestive of inflammatory back pain, I would refer the patient directly to a rheumatologist who can then arrange whichever investigations seem appropriate.

Should HLA-B27 be looked for routinely?

- No. When the clinical suspicion of inflammatory back pain is high, this test may help to confirm the diagnosis.

Management
General

Early diagnosis of inflammatory back pain is of the essence if treatment is to have the best chance of preventing permanent stiffness and deformity. Patient education is of prime importance and the sooner this is started, the better. It is important that the patient understands the difference between inflammatory and simple back pain as they are more likely to comply with treatments such as non-steroidal anti-inflammatory drugs (NSAIDs) and physiotherapy. The patient should also be made aware of other complications of spondyloarthropathy. In particular, the risk of acute anterior uveitis should be clearly explained together with the need for an emergency visit to an ophthalmologist in such a case. The patient should be advised not to smoke because chest expansion may become limited. I often advise patients with AS to join the National Ankylosing Spondylitis Society (NASS), and there are other self-help groups for patients with other conditions.

Exercise

Physiotherapy, in conjunction with an appropriate NSAID, is the mainstay of treatment for inflammatory back pain. Patients with AS in particular, should be taught a daily exercise regime that should become as routine as brushing their teeth. Lying prone for a short period every day (perhaps for 15 minutes whilst watching television) is a good habit to get into. Swimming is an excellent form of exercise which encourages back extension. Generally, I advise patients to avoid contact sports such as rugby, but in practice there is little that I would stop someone doing if they were keen to continue.

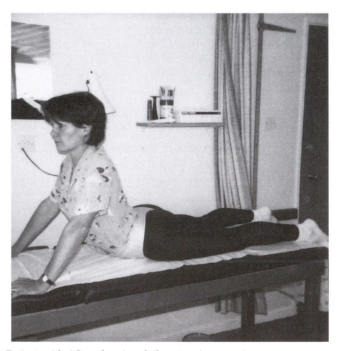

Figure 7.2 Patient with AS performing daily extension exercises.

Non-steroidal anti-inflammatory drugs

Patients with inflammatory back pain respond very well to NSAIDs, which is often another feature that distinguishes this group of patients from those with mechanical back pain. An emerging question is whether the spondyloarthropathies, in particular AS, have become less severe since the introduction and the long-term use of NSAIDs.

Many NSAIDs have been shown to be useful in the treatment of AS,[13] but it is impossible to predict which NSAID will be both efficient and well tolerated. It is often therefore a case of 'trial and error' to find which particular drug suits which individual patient best. I tend to use a slow-release preparation such as diclofenac 75 mg b.d. but would use up to 100 mg b.d. if necessary. This helps to ease early morning stiffness, enabling the patient to get going and to do their exercises. Phenylbutazone is still used by hospital consultants for the treatment of AS (on a named-patient basis) when other NSAIDs do not work.

Second-line drugs

There has been much debate about whether second-line drugs are useful for the treatment of axial disease in the spondyloarthropathies. Sulphasalazine is of use when there is peripheral arthritis[14] but probably has no effect on axial disease progression.[15] No other second-line drugs have been sufficiently studied to know whether they are of use or not.

Systemic corticosteroids have no place in the routine treatment of the spondyloarthropathies – they do not influence the progression of the disease process and their chronic use is associated with unwanted side effects. Occasionally, when NSAIDs are ineffective, even at high doses, it may be appropriate to give 'pulsed' therapy with methylprednisolone.

Summary

- The diagnosis of inflammatory back pain is dependent largely on the clinical history and examination
- The modified Schober's test is the most useful examination technique in the surgery.
- Investigations, including blood tests and X-rays, are usually normal early in the course of the disease.
- HLA-B27 should not be looked for routinely but may help to confirm the diagnosis.
- Patient education is very important.
- Physiotherapy and exercise together with NSAIDs are the main-stay of treatment.
- High doses of NSAIDs may need to be used.

References

1. Dougados, M., van der Linden, S., Juhlin, R. *et al.* (1991). The European Study Group preliminary criteria for the classification of spondyloarthropathy. *Arthritis Rheum.*, **34**,1218–1227.
2. Zeidler, H., Mau, W. and Khan, M.A. (1992). Undifferentiated spondyloarthropathies. *Rheum. Dis. Clin. North Am.*, **18**, 187–202.
3. Braun, J., Bollow, M., Remlinger, G. *et al.* (1998). Prevalence of spondyloarthropathies in HLA-B27 positive and negative blood donors. *Arthritis Rheum.*, **41**, 58–67.
4. McCormick, A., Fleming, D. and Charlton, J. (1995). *Morbidity Statistics from General Practice. Fourth National Study* 1991–1992. HMSO.
5. Hodgkin, K. (1985). *Towards Earlier Diagnosis*. 5th edn. Churchill Livingstone.
6. Underwood, M.R. and Dawes, P. (1995). Inflammatory back pain in primary care. *Br. J. Rheumatol.*, **34**, 1074–1077.

7. Calin, A., Porta, J., Fries, J.F. and Schurman, D.J. (1977). Clinical history as a screening test for ankylosing spondylitis. *JAMA*, **237**, 2613–2614.
8. Jenkinson, T.R., Mallorie, P.A., Whitelock, H.C., Kennedy, L.G., Garrett, S.L. and Calin, A. (1994). Defining spinal mobility in ankylosing spondylitis (AS). The Bath AS Metrology Index. *J. Rheumatol.*, **21**, 1694–1698.
9. McKay, K., Brophy, S., Mack, C. *et al.* (1997). Patterns of radiological axial involvement in 470 ankylosing spondylitis patients (abstract). *Arthritis Rheum.*, **40**(Suppl.), 61.
10. Battistone, M., Manaster, B.J., Reda, D.J. *et al.* (1997). Patterns of sacroiliitis among the spondyloarthropathies: Analysis of data from a large multicenter cohort (abstract). *Arthritis Rheum.*, **40**(Suppl.), 65.
11. Braun, J., Bollow, M. and Sieper, J. (1998). Radiologic diagnosis and pathology of the spondyloarthropathies. *Rheum. Dis. Clin. North Am.*, **24**, 697–735.
12. Hawkins, B.R., Dawkins, R.L., Christiansen, F.T. and Zilko, P.J. (1981). Use of the B27 test in the diagnosis of ankylosing spondylitis: a statistical evaluation. *Arthritis Rheum.*, **24**, 743–746.
13. Rosenbloom, D., Brooks, P., Bellamy, N. and Buchanan, W. (1985). *Clinical Trials in the Rheumatic Diseases: A Selected Critical Review.* Praeger, pp. 262–279.
14. Kirwan, J., Edwards, A., Huitfeldt, B. *et al.* (1993).The course of established ankylosing spondylitis and the effects of sulphasalazine over 3 years. *Br. J. Rheumatol.*, **32**, 729.
15. Taylor, H.G., Beswick, E.J., and Dawes, P.T. (1991). Sulphasalazine in ankylosing spondylitis. A radiological, clinical and laboratory assessment. *Clin. Rheumatol.*, **10**, 43.

Chapter 8

Neoplasms of the Spine

Tom Cadoux-Hudson

Introduction

Neoplasia of the spine is rare but the presentation is often insidious and symptoms can easily be confused with less serious conditions affecting the spine. The GP is therefore confronted with the quintessential primary care challenge of distinguishing between common musculoskeletal disorders that cause low back and neck pain and the very much rarer myelopathies from spinal cord compression.

The slow onset may be due to the spinal cord's ability to accommodate slow compression, producing 'compression paraplegia'. The initial symptoms of spinal cord compression can be mild, with trivial mid-line spine discomfort combined with slight functional loss and soft sensory symptoms such as tingling and numbness. The final presentation however may be rapid, relentless loss of function associated with poor outcomes.

Early diagnosis with appropriate intervention is associated with better outcomes. The combination of these factors has put a greater emphasis on careful clinical selection and early appropriate investigation. The purpose of this chapter is to describe our current knowledge of epidemiology, causes and presentation of neoplasia of the spine to enable early diagnosis.

The most robust classification system for neoplasia of the spine considers extradural and intradural tumours, of which extradural is more common. The intradural tumours sub-divide into extramedullary and intramedullary, with extramedullary causes representing 80 per cent. This classification system was initially developed when myelography was the gold standard diagnostic tool. However this classification remains clinically robust in the magnetic resonance imaging era. A number of other factors are also important including the direction from which the compression is coming from; susceptibility to ischaemia between grey and white matter; speed of compression.

Classification

Extradural (common)

Usually metastases or haemopoietic neoplasms such as myeloma, lymphoma, leukaemia deposits or plastacytoma

Intradural (less common)

80% extra-medullary
20% intra-medullary

Incidence

Accurate epidemiology describing spinal cord neoplasia is lacking, particularly for intramedullary neoplasia. The extramedullary tumours are largely caused by metastatic and haemopoietic neoplasia. The intradural/extramedullary tumours are due predominantly to neurofibromas and meningiomas. The intramedullary tumours present with a mean age of 40 years but are represented in all ages, and affect the sexes equally.[1,2]

Pathology

Extramedullary neoplasia

The extramedullary neoplasia is usually metastatic disease from the common primary sites such as breast, prostate, lung and less commonly, renal and bowel. The predilection of breast, prostate and lung for spreading to the vertebral bodies may be related to the high blood flow through these remaining haemopoietic sites or changes in venous drainage induced by the primary tumour.

These secondaries usually start in the vertebral bodies with destruction of softer cancellous bone followed by cortical bone resulting in rapid collapse, anterior spinal artery and cord compression. Spinal cord infarction often follows vertebral body collapse. However the epidural space may be initially involved, allowing for a more gradual cord compression and a lower incidence of spinal cord infarction. Involvement of the vertebral body pedicles and neural arch follows rapidly. Disruption of the facet joints will accelerate instability.

The blood supply of the spinal cord may also be involved early. The spinal cord receives its blood supply from a few critical points; the anterior spinal artery starts from the vertebral artery at the craniocervical junction and supplies the cervical spinal cord. However radicular arteries at the cervicothoracic and lower thorax are essential for adequate nutrient supply. Metastatic disease at T11/12 (origin of the artery of Adam Kiewicz) and the cervicothoracic junction may cause an anterior spinal infarct with minimal cord compression.

The rarer extradural tumours include chordomas (remnants related to the notochord), osteoid-related tumours, haemopoietic tumours such as myeloma, lymphoma, plasmacytoma and leukaemia deposits.

Extramedullary

The commonest tumours causing extramedullary compression are neurofibroma and meningioma. Neurofibroma may be isolated primaries or part of von Recklinghausen's disease (Neurofibromatosis Type I rather than type II). Neurofibromata start within the exiting nerve root, usually the sensory nerve rootlet. The fibrous cells, of spindle shape, spread for a short distance along the nerve and exit through the adjacent foramina giving a characteristic 'dumb-bell' shape. These slow-growing tumours can reach considerable size within the chest or abdominal cavity before diagnosis. Meningioma are usually seen in women, grow very slowly and are solitary. Occasional dysraphic or developmental anomalies present as extramedullary fibrolipomatous deposits. Spinal bifida occulta may be associated with these anomalies.

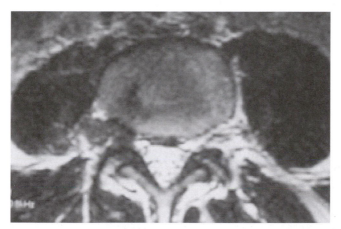

Figure 8.1 Neurofibroma compressing the L4 nerve and partly affecting the L3 far laterally at the L3/4 level. Removed with some nerve root without neurological loss. Presented with wasting of the right thigh preceded by anterior knee pain.

Intramedullary

The intramedullary tumours are mainly derived from the common cells found maintaining and supporting the central nervous system (CNS). They usually arise from the cervical and upper thoracic spinal cord. Ependymomas (37 per cent) arise from ependymal cells which line the internal cerebrospinal fluid channels (ventricles and spinal canal). As a result ependymomas can spread through the CNS, with up to 40 per cent arising from primaries in the posterior fossa. Astrocytoma (24 per cent) arise from astrocytes and are more commonly seen in children and may be aggressive infiltrating tumours, rarely spreading through the dura mater.

Vascular tumours (11 per cent) represent the next largest group, with haemangioblastomas and cavernomas the commonest of these. Haemangioblastomas may be solitary or multiple as part of von Hippel-Lindau (VHL) disease (autosomal recessive), with retina and renal involvement.

Developmental related intramedullary tumours include epidermoids and dermoids arising from skin cell arrests continuing to deposit keratin (epidermoids) or adnexal deposits (sebum, keratin etc).

Symptoms

The patient may present with mild and progressive, if not intermittent, symptoms. Pain, usually mid-line, aching in nature, exacerbated by movement may precede functional symptoms. At the early stage there may be little to distinguish neoplastic mid-line pain from the far more common musculoskeletal and degenerative causes. Mid-line pain can also occur with nerve root pain.

Pain

Mid-line spinal pain caused by spinal neoplasia usually develops a characteristic pattern. Initially this aching discomfort is indistinguishable from other more common causes. However as the spinal cord becomes compressed a diurnal variation may develop, with the night being the worst time.

Musculoskeletal degenerative pain may also occur at night, but neoplastic pain may drive the patient out of bed. Degenerative pain is usually relieved by changing posture in bed. The neoplastic pain patient will get up and pace about, make a cup of tea, taking some more analgesia. They may return to bed and sleep a few more hours before being woken and arising from bed again. Some will prefer to sleep sitting up in a chair.

This diurnal type of mid-line aching pain associated with a previous history of a histologically proven primary neoplasm elsewhere should be considered due to a metastasis until proved otherwise.

Neoplasia of the spine may also involve the nearby nerve roots causing a typical brachialgia with sharp stabbing pains radiating down the relevant dermatome and myotome. This distribution may be indistinguishable from brachialgia caused by intervertebral disc prolapse or osteophyte disease.

Nerve root pain is typically episodic and words such as shooting, stabbing and burning are often used, usually spreading along a dermatomal or occasionally a deeper 'myotomal' route. Numbness may be experienced between bouts of pain.

Segmental pathology, intramedullary lesions, can produce a 'central' pain, aching in nature which has a diffuse distribution, such as a girdle distribution with thoracic lesions. Lhermitte described this 'central' pain associated with bouts of body tingling in extremes of neck flexion and extension where the diameter of the cervical cord is reduced and spinal cord moves with respect to the canal.

Functional loss

Spinal cord compression can produce predominantly motor symptoms such as weakness, loss of facility and clumsiness. These symptoms are often due to anterior spinal column compression, typically from vertebral body metastasis. Upper motor neuron compression typically causes clumsiness or loss of facility; difficulty with fine movements such as writing and holding cups and saucers. Loss of power may occur late in the upper limbs. High cervical cord compression can also produce a peculiar diffuse wasting of the small muscles of the hands.

The lower limbs develop a pyramidal type of weakness with weakness of the hip flexors/extensors before weakness of dorsiflexors. The patient will report difficulty getting up stairs and rising from a chair. Partners may have to 'push' the patient up the stairs. The patient may walk with 'stiff' legs, catching uneven paving stones.

Loss of bladder control occurs late in progressive spinal cord compression. Incontinence develops as the patient becomes unable to weight bear and sensory loss spreads.

Sensory loss usually occurs later, but tingling or 'pins and needles', typical nervous system complaints, may occur early. The cervical spine neoplastic compression may generate 'electric shocks' on neck movement; Lhermitte's sign. Coughing can have a similar effect. Ascending sensory loss is usually a late symptom.

Signs

Upper motor neuron (UMN) signs; hypertonia, hyper-reflexia and weakness without muscle wasting are typically present, but rarely without symptoms. If nerve root involvement is present the UMN signs may be reduced by lower motor neuron (LMN) pathology; a LMN lesion 'trumps' a UMN lesion. This phenomena is a particular problem in the cervical region and can 'mask' UMN signs in the upper limbs.

In the lower limbs proximal muscle weakness is associated with 'up going' plantar responses. Care should be taken not to evoke a pain withdrawal response by using sharp objects such as car keys. This will produce a false-positive plantar response, as will tickling the sole of the foot. The adductor reflex appears with UMN lesions.

The abdominal reflexes, elicited by diagonal stroking of the abdominal quadrants, will be absent with mid-thoracic and higher lesions.

Sensory abnormalities will initially be patchy, forming clear 'levels' as cord compression becomes complete. The sacrum is usually spared. Touch, as opposed to pain elicited by a sharp object (pin is often the favoured weapon) is often the first dorsal column function to be affected. Touch varies in different surfaces (hair bearing; flexor; extensor) but most patients have a clear perception of how touch should feel. Compare one limb with another. Compare sensation on the affected limb with the face etc.

Sensation is a subjective finding and anxious patients can occasionally be unreliable witnesses. This source of error can be reduced by starting from insensate areas and working towards regions of normality.

Lateral compression of the spinal cord (Brown-Séquard syndrome) will produce a dissociated sensory loss, with reduction of ipsilateral dorsal column function (touch) and reduction in contralateral spinothalamic (temperature) sensation. This can be elicited from the history, particularly in the UK where patients are fond of baths rather than showers. The patients may report that the bath water, which felt 'normal' to the feet burns their buttocks on sitting down in the bath. Hands may get burnt with matches without generating pain. A Brown-Séquard syndrome can precede significant motor weakness.

Table 8.1 Red flags.

Pain	Nocturnal pain	Waking at night after a few hours sleep Getting out of bed Pacing about Returning to sleep; to wake again a few hours later
	Lhermitte's sign	'Central' pain Diffuse tingling with flexion/extension of the neck
Cervical syndromes	High cervical compression (C1–3)	Occasional trigeminal involvement and nystagmus Occipital/nape of neck pain Diffuse small muscle wasting in hands Brisk deltoid reflexes/no jaw jerk; UMN signs in upper + lower limbs Lhermitte's sign
	Mid-cervical (C4–5)	No deltoid reflex, deltoid wasting Weakness Brisk triceps; biceps reflex may be absent UMN in lower limbs Abdominal reflex absent Plantars 'up-going' Ascending sensory level Lhermitte's sign
	Lower cervical (C6–8)	Normal or absent biceps/triceps Finger jerk Absent abdominal reflexes UMN in lower limbs Lhermitte's sign Pain 'between shoulder blades'
Thoracic syndromes		Absent abdominal reflexes Pain Sensory level
Lumbar (conus) syndromes		Nerve root; 'femoralgia' and 'sciatica' Sacral numbness, early bladder disturbance Brisk ankle reflex with absent knee reflex; abdominal reflex present

In the elderly unilateral weakness from spinal cord compression will need to be differentiated from cerebrovascular accidents (CVA) which usually involve the face (brachiofacial). Acute painless paraparesis is usually due to anterior spinal artery infarct which can be spontaneous or more rarely related to neoplasia. Acute onset of spinal cord compression will produce dramatic functional loss with no significant UMN signs due to 'spinal shock'. Several days may have to elapse before UMN signs appear. This can make spinal cord compression in the confused and unco-operative a difficult diagnosis.

Investigations

Whilst plain X-rays do not have a useful role in degenerative diseases of the spinal column, they still have a use where spinal column neoplasia is considered to be involved. A patient with typical night-time spinal pain, a previous history of neoplastic primary, and mild UMN signs may achieve a clear diagnosis on plain X-rays. Chest X-rays will help establish whether secondary disease has developed elsewhere and help exclude patients unsuitable for general anaesthetic where 'cannon-ball' secondaries will cause lung collapse.

Magnetic resonance imaging (MRI) has become the most accurate way of investigating spinal cord neoplasia, providing excellent resolution of spinal cord, nerve roots, cerebrospinal fluid (CSF) but with limited resolution of bony structures. However few MRI scanners can accurately image the whole spine in one 'session', a service provided by traditional myelography. With a clear history and strong crisp clinical signs a 'single' level MRI (cervical, thoracic, lumbar) may be appropriate. However the whole spine may have to be imaged if the history and clinical signs are not clear. Neuro-axis MRI is also required if the identified lesion may be an intramedullary/conus lesion suggesting ependymoma or astrocytoma to exclude distant CNS primaries. Whole spine MRI has the disadvantages of either reduced resolution or excessive MRI time; or both. A normal 'single level' MRI does not exclude pathology elsewhere in the spinal column. MRI is not as sensitive as classical isotope bone scanning for identifying intravertebral metastasis.

Computerized tomography (CT) scanning as a primary investigation for spinal column neoplasia is not helpful, and should be reserved for specialist centre use when resolving bony stability prior to surgery. However where MRI is not available, or contraindicated, CT scanning as an adjunct to myelography is a reasonable alternative. Contraindications include cardiac pacemaker, MRI incompatible aneurysm clips (used after aneurysmal subarachnoid haemorrhage) or magnetic metallic objects (shrapnel etc).

Treatment

Non-surgical treatment is appropriate where the patient has a well-recognized primary, multiple metastatic disease and generalized ill health. The appropriate management involves palliative pain relief, regional radiotherapy and chemotherapy if indicated. Single dose external beam radiotherapy is an effective and fast way of controlling relentless mid-line spinal column pain. Non-steroidal anti-inflammatories (NSAID's) are also surprisingly effective. Opiate analgesics tend to produce drowsiness and disorientation, with increasing doses required for long-term pain control.

Surgical treatment is required to establish the diagnosis, tumour bulk reduction/removal where appropriate, and spinal column stabilization where possible. Biopsy can be achieved under local anaesthetic (LA) with CT scan guidance, with variable accuracy (60–90%) rate depending on the 'toughness' of the tumour and accessibility. Failure of LA biopsy should be followed by open biopsy under general anaesthetic (GA).

Few extradural metastatic tumours can be entirely removed. The main aim of surgery is to achieve spinal/nerve root decompression and stabilization. Intradural extramedullary tumours can be removed where the nerve roots are not critically involved. Extramedullary tumours of the conus region can be removed but compromise is occasionally required to

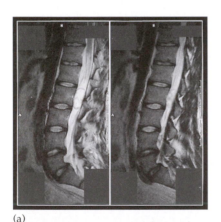

(a)

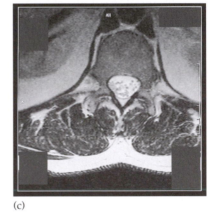

(c)

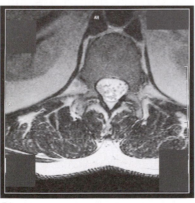

(b)

Figure 8.2 MRI showing ependymoma.
(a) Sagittal view. (b) Axial view.
(c) Axial view of normal level for comparison.

preserve bladder and lower limb function. Intramedullary tumours such as astrocytomas are rarely completely resectable, despite advances in pre-operative imaging and resection techniques.

Prognosis

Extradural tumours

Metastatic spread from the prostate and breast carries a better prognosis in term of morbidity and mortality than renal, bowel and lung primaries. The rate of progression of the spinal cord compression tends to be slower and adjuvant therapy (hormonal and chemotherapy) tends to be more effective in controlling disease progression. As a result it is more appropriate to carry out extensive decompression and reconstructive surgery for breast and prostate disease. Biopsy and radiotherapy may be a suitable alternative to aggressive decompressive/reconstructive surgery in lung and renal spinal column secondary treatment.

Extramedullary

Primary resection of these tumours is the treatment of choice. Reconstructive stabilization of the spinal column is rarely required except at the craniocervical junction. Complete resection achieves the best long-term results. Complete resection may not be possible in the conus region and with certain developmental tumours such as epidermoids and dermoids. Repeated resections may be more appropriate where bladder function is at major risk.

Intramedullary

The majority of these tumours cannot be completely resected. The outcome is largely dependent on the pre-operative status and whether resection was achieved.[1] However the reports detailing recovery after surgery are few, the pathology heterogeneous and numbers of patients small.

Astrocytomas usually recur within 1–2 years of primary resection and can spread elsewhere in the CNS; mortality can be expected to be 25 per cent at 2 years. Ependymomas can be remarkably radiosensitive and more amenable to complete resection; 85 per cent of patients alive at 5 years. Haemangioblastomas and cavernoma are also amenable to resection. In VHL, multiple lesions can make surgery a palliative procedure.

Summary

Neoplasia of the spine is a relatively rare condition but the consequences of delay in diagnosis and treatment are considerable to the patient. The diagnostic difficulties are further exacerbated by the high incidence of benign mid-line spine pain particularly in the lumbar region. The role of accurate history taking, clinical examination and awareness of a few 'red flags' will greatly assist in the selection and timing of patients for further investigation and treatment.

References

1. Cooper, P. (1989). Outcome after operative treatment of intramedullary spinal cord tumours in adults: Intermediate and long term results in 51 patients. *Neurosurgery,* **25,** 855–9.
2. Cristante, L and Herrman, H.D. (1994). Surgical management of intramedullary spinal cord tumours: functional outcome and sources of morbidity. *Neurosurgery,* **35,** 69–76.

Chapter 9

Spinal Infection

Andrew Wainwright

Introduction

Spinal infection is an unusual but important cause of back pain with a reported incidence of paralysis in up to 50 per cent of patients.[1] Before the antibiotic era, mortality was between 40–70% and even now it is estimated to be 1–20%, depending on the organism. Recent advances with aggressive diagnosis and treatment have altered the natural history and improved the prognosis.

The current problems with spinal infections are the delay in diagnosis (averaging 3 months), the long recovery period (averaging 12 months)[1] and the great cost of treatment.

In most cases the history contains 'red flag' symptoms,[2] including rest pain, night pain, night sweats and general malaise.

The overall aims of treatment are to eradicate infection and prevent neurological deficit, spinal instability or deformity.

Pyogenic vertebral osteomyelitis

A survey in Denmark[3] found an incidence of five cases of acute vertebral osteomyelitis per million of population per year. The highest incidence was between 60–69 years (18 per million per year). There has been a recent increase in the incidence in general and particularly between 20–29 years old which may reflect a population with drug abuse. Males are more commonly affected (55–75%).

Unremitting pain is characteristic,[4] which may be vague, non-specific, and without dermatomal or radicular pattern. Often there is a predisposing source of bacteraemia, such as pneumonia, urinary tract infection, skin infection. Diabetes or immunological compromise is a risk factor. Local spinal tenderness is often but not always present, spasm and loss of motion are seen. Fever is present in about half of cases.

Neurological deficits are seen in 17–40% of cases, especially in older patients, those with infections at higher levels in the spine (i.e. cervical), other debilitating disease (e.g. diabetes, rheumatoid), and in those with significant delay in diagnosis. This may be due to compression from pus, bone, disc or granulomatous tissue.

The lumbar spine is most commonly affected (50 per cent of cases), followed by the thoracic spine. The cervical spine is involved in fewer than 10 per cent of cases. Paraspinal soft tissues are commonly involved but frank abscesses are not always seen. Presentation may be variable. Four types of clinical syndrome have been described[5] and are shown in Table 9.1.

Table 9.1 Four types of clinical syndrome

Abdominal syndrome	– with symptoms and signs suggestive of peritonitis.
Hip joint syndrome	– with acute pain in the hip, flexion contracture and decreased range of movement.
Meningeal syndrome	– suggestive of acute suppurative or TB meningitis.
Back pain syndrome	– onset may be acute or insidious.

Although *Staphylococcus aureus* was historically the exclusive pathogen, it now accounts for only 50 per cent[6] and organisms are often multiply resistant. Other causal organisms are Gram-negative bacteria (*E.coli, Enterococcus, Proteus*) and *Pseudomonas*, the latter is often isolated in intravenous drug abusers.

Urgent investigation of these patients is necessary once clinical suspicion has been raised. Diagnosis via blood cultures is only positive in 24 per cent. White blood count is elevated in only 42 per cent of individuals, the erythrocyte sedimentation rate (ESR) is high in 90 per cent. The CRP (an acute phase protein) is usually raised and can be used as a more accurate measure of clinical response. A rapid decrease in the ESR during the first month of treatment represents success; however persistently raised ESR does not mean failure and one should rely on clinical signs and CRP.

Although characteristic changes may be seen on radiographs, these do not occur until at least two weeks from onset. A 'normal x-ray' may give a false sense of security. Magnetic resonance imaging (MRI) is the most useful imaging investigation as it is both sensitive for detecting infection (96 per cent) and specific[7] for differentiating infection from other conditions, including tumour (specificity 93 per cent, accuracy 94 per cent). However, it is less good for monitoring progress as it lags behind the clinical situation and it remains abnormal while other clinical indicators return to normal.[8]

Tissue diagnosis by blood cultures or aspirate of the infection (e.g. by computerized tomography (CT)-guided needle biopsy) is mandatory. For neurologically intact patients, the treatment of choice is a 6–12 week course of antibiotics and immobilization, using bed rest, followed by bracing. Use of antibiotics before biopsy will decrease the chance of isolating the causal organism. Open biopsy may be required and further surgery may be necessary in order to debride refractory cases, drain abscesses, or prevent neurological deterioration, bone destruction or deformity.

Disc space infection in children

Osteomyelitis of the vertebral end plates may secondarily invade the disc space, particularly in children. *Staphylococcus aureus* is the most common identified organism, however an organism is not identified in every case. Gram-negative bacteria are common in older patients. Children of any age (mean age, 7 years) commonly present with the inability to walk, stand or sit and complain of back pain or tenderness.[7] Physical findings are of spinal tenderness, decreased range of movement, malaise and irritability; they may also hold themselves erect. Neurological abnormalities are unusual, but if present are ominous. Diagnosis is frequently delayed.

Blood tests may be normal except for an elevated white blood count and ESR. Radiographs show characteristic changes, but these do not occur until 10 days from onset. MRI scans are the best diagnostic tool; suggestive in 90 per cent of individuals. Treatment includes bed rest and immobilization. Antibiotics are used when there is a positive biopsy. Most children are

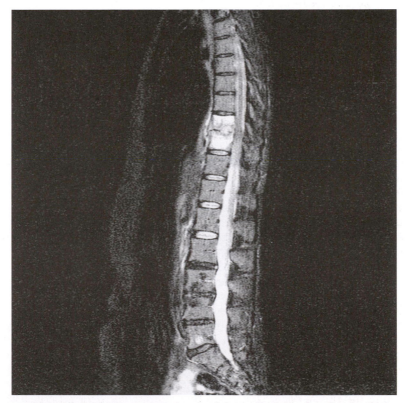

Figure 9.1 Sagittal magnetic resonance image of thoracolumbar spine, showing high signal within the vertebral bodies of T9 and T10 and paravertebral extension, with destruction of the disc in between them. Note the different appearance of this area of discitis compared to the areas of degenerative changes in the lower lumbar area.

asymptomatic after this. Spontaneous fusion occurs in 25 per cent of cases. They rarely require surgery and long-term low back pain is rare.

The incidence of disc space infection in adults is most commonly secondary to surgery. Rates after disc surgery range from 1–2.8% and after discography, 1 per cent. Prophylactic antibiotics probably reduce these incidences. The diagnosis is made with a history of back pain, muscle spasm, and difficulty walking following spinal instrumentation. The ESR and CRP (which should be back to normal within 4 weeks of spinal surgery) will be raised.[9] Disc space biopsy by open or closed methods before antibiotics are given will identify an organism in over 50 per cent of cases and treatment should continue until the CRP is normal.

Spinal tuberculosis (TB, Pott's disease)

This was first described by Hippocrates in the fourth century BC, although evidence for deformity attributable to TB has been found in the spines of Egyptian mummies and Neolithic remains up to 7000 BC. However, it was Percival Pott, the English surgeon, who gave the first full report of this condition in 1779.

TB is prevalent in underdeveloped countries. It is increasing in the developed world with increased immunosuppression (e.g. with AIDS, chemotherapy and transplantation). The spine is the most common extrapleural site. It may spread along the longitudinal ligament and cause destruction of several contiguous spinal levels or result in skip lesions (15 per cent) or abscess formation. This diagnosis should not be forgotten in otherwise fit adults in the UK.

Individuals are chronically ill and have pain, weight loss, malaise and night sweats. In the later stages, there may be deformity or paraplegia secondary to neural compression. The thoracolumbar spine is most commonly affected; the cervical spine and sacro-iliac joints are rarely affected. It may present with a psoas abscess (pain on passive extension of the hip, stretching the psoas). Other findings are similar to vertebral osteomyelitis. Severe kyphosis, sinus formation or (Pott's) paraplegia are late sequelae.

About two-thirds of patients have abnormal chest X-rays. Twenty per cent have a negative skin test for TB. The ESR is raised,[10] though white counts may be normal. The imaging modality of choice is MRI although characteristic changes may be seen on plain radiographs.

Specimens taken from microbiological culture are positive in 50 per cent of cases and may take 16 weeks to show a result. More modern techniques of polymerase chain reaction (PCR) are reported to have a sensitivity of 95 per cent, and an accuracy of 92 per cent.[11]

Epidural space infections

Epidural abscesses are becoming more common as the number of spinal procedures increases. It is a medical and surgical emergency. The mortality of this condition is still 20 per cent.

The condition presents with severe, intractable back pain in 94 per cent of cases, with fever and tenderness. Without treatment, this will progress to radicular pain, weakness, and eventually paralysis. However, the diagnosis is often delayed owing to the variable presentation.

Blood cultures are positive in 60 per cent of individuals. *Staphylococcus aureus* is responsible for over 60 per cent of cases and Gram-negative rods for 20 per cent. Lumbar puncture is not to be performed as this risks meningitis and neurological deterioration. Mortality prior to antibiotics was 50 per cent. The prognosis now, with aggressive surgical decompression, is recovery in 78 per cent. It is optimal if treated within 36 hours of onset. Poor prognostic factors include age, HIV, diabetes, neurological deficit, complete loss of sensation, rapid paralysis lasting more than 36 hours, or acute paralysis within 12 hours, (indicative of cord ischaemia or infarction).

Brucellosis

This is found mostly in farm and abattoir workers and vets, having been transmitted from dogs and farm animals. The organism, which is found in dogs and farm animals, causes non-caseating Gram-negative lesions. Symptoms include polyarthralgia, fever, night-sweats and anorexia. Brucella titres of greater than 1:80 are diagnostic. These can often recur after treatment.

Differential diagnosis

The differential diagnosis of spinal infection includes primary and secondary malignancy, metabolic bone disease, rheumatoid arthritis, ankylosing spondylitis, or infection of soft tissues and related organs of the hip, abdomen and genito-urinary system.

Summary

- Pain is the most common presenting feature.
- The 'red flag' symptoms and signs are often positive for this serious condition and should initiate prompt referral (less than 4 weeks) and urgent MRI.
- These symptoms and signs include particularly:
  - presentation less than 20 years or over 55 years
  - non-mechanical, or rest pain
  - thoracic pain
  - associated use of steroids, IV drug abuse/HIV
  - malaise, weight loss
  - night sweats or fever (although temperature elevation may be minimal)
  - neurological deficit or paralysis.

- The most common sign is localized tenderness and sustained paravertebral spasm with decreased range of movement of the spine.
- Prompt diagnosis and management can reduce serious morbidity or even mortality.

References

1. Wood, G.W. II. (1998). Infections of spine. In *Campbell's Operative Orthopaedics* (S. Terry Canale, ed.) pp. 3094–3124, Mosby Year Book.
2. RCGP. (1996). Clinical Guidelines for the Management of Acute Low Back Pain. Royal College of General Practitioners. Website – http://www.rcgp.org.uk
3. Krogsgard, M.R., Wagn, P., and Bengtsson, J. (1998). Epidemiology of acute vertebral osteomyelitis in Denmark. *Acta Orthop. Scand.*, **69**, 513–517.
4. Carragee, E.J. (1997). Pyogenic vertebral osteomyelitis. *J. Bone Joint Surg.*, **79**(A), 874–880.
5. Puig-Guri, J. (1946). Pyogenic osteomyelitis of the spine: differential diagnosis through clinical and roentgenographic observations. *J. Bone Joint Surg.*, **28**, 28–39.
6. Sapico, F.L. (1996). Microbiology and antimicrobial therapy of spinal infections. *Orthop. Clin. North Am.*, **27**, 9–13
7. Wisneski, R.J. (1991). Infectious disease of the spine. *Orthop. Clin. North Am.*, **22**, 491–501.
8. Carragee, E.J. (1997). The clinical use of magnetic resonance imaging in pyogenic vertebral osteomyelitis. *Spine*, **22**, 780–785.
9. Thelander, U. and Larsson, S. (1992). Quantitation of C-reactive protein levels and erythrocyte sedimentation rate after spinal surgery. *Spine*, **17**, 400–403.
10. Boachie-Adjei, O. and Sequillante, R.G. (1996). Tuberculosis of the spine. *Orthop. Clin. North Am.*, **27**, 95–103.
11. Berk, R.H., Yazici, M., Atabey, N. *et al.* (1996). Detection of *Mycobacterium tuberculosis* in formaldehyde solution-fixed, paraffin embedded tissue by polymerase chain reaction in Pott's disease. *Spine*, **21**, 1991–1995.

Chapter 10

Metabolic Disorders of the Spine

Roger Smith

Introduction

Bone is a metabolically active tissue which is constantly being removed and replaced. It is composed of an organic matrix, mainly collagen, upon which is deposited a mineral phase of complex calcium salts known as hydroxyapatite.[1] 'Classic' metabolic bone diseases which affect both components include osteoporosis, osteomalacia, Paget's disease and parathyroid disease (Table 1). In addition there are many rare disorders of the skeleton mainly due to defective synthesis of the organic components of bone which can be regarded as 'new' metabolic bone diseases. The physician should be able to recognize these if only to refer them for specialist advice. Osteoporosis and Paget's disease are the commonest metabolic diseases affecting the spine.

Table 10.1 Metabolic bone diseases and the spine

Disease	Effect on the spine	Comments
Classic		
Osteoporosis	Vertebral collapse, irregular wedging, loss of height	Exclude secondary causes
Paget's disease	Vertebral deformity and enlargement	Nerve compression common
Osteomalacia	Regular biconcavity	Rarely cord compression due to enthesiopathy
Parathyroid bone disease	Sclerosis and porosis	Very rarely brown tumour
New		
Osteogenesis imperfecta	Kyphoscoliosis in severe forms	
Chondrodysplasias Achondroplasia	Various structural changes Narrow interpedicular distance	Abnormal cervical spine Cord and root compression worse if thoracolumbar deformity
Marfan's syndrome	Scoliosis	
Alkaptonuria	Calcification of intervertebral discs	Ochronosis

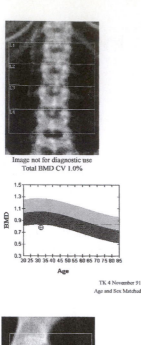

Image not for diagnostic use
Total BMD CV 1.0%

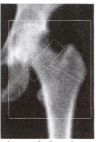

TK 4 November 91
Age and Sex Matched

(A)

Scan Information:

Scan:	16-Mar-00 - A0316000A
Scan Mode:	Fast Performance
Analysis:	16-Mar-00 12:28 - Ver 8.26
Operator:	JR
Model:	Hologic QDR-4000 (S/N 55045)
Comment:	ECR

Region	Area [cm²]	BMC [g]	BMD [g/cm²]
L1	10.85	7.05	0.650
L2	12.26	9.33	0.761
L3	13.71	11.38	0.830
L4	16.44	13.69	0.833
Total	53.26	41.45	0.778

Results Summary:

Total BMD:		0.778 g/cm²	
Peak reference:	74%	T score:	-2.4
Age matched:	75%	Z score:	-2.4

Physician Comments:

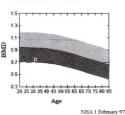

Image not for diagnostic use
Total BMD CV 1.0%

NHA 1 February 97
Age and Sex Matched

(B)

Scan Information:

Scan:	16-Mar-00 - A0316000B
Scan Mode:	Fast Performance
Analysis:	16-Mar-00 12:35 - Ver 8.26
Operator:	JR
Model:	Hologic QDR-4000 (S/N 55045)
Comment:	ECR

Region	Area [cm²]	BMC [g]	BMD [g/cm²]
Neck	5.79	4.04	0.699
Trochanter	9.97	5.49	0.551
Inter	20.86	17.68	0.847
Total	36.62	27.21	0.743
Ward's	1.07	0.60	0.563

Results Summary:

Total[L] BMD:		0.743 g/cm²	
Peak reference:	79%	T score:	-1.6
Age matched:	79%	Z score:	-1.6

Physician Comment:

Figure 10.1 Bone density charts of a 32-year-old woman. Areas covered are L1 to L4 (chart A) and the hip (chart B). Images are included on the charts to ensure there are no gross abnormalities. The density print out is shown below each image. The normal range (mean=2 standard deviations) is given in the boxes. You can see that normally bone density in women falls from about age 40. The result from the patient is measured as bone mineral density (BMD) and expressed in relation to the mean as standard deviations below or above. Where it is compared with peak bone mass, the standard deviations are expressed as T score. Where it is expressed in relation to mean for age, the result is expressed as a Z score. In this case the results for T and Z scores are the same. The low T (and Z) score of 2.4 is defined as osteopenia (-1 to -2.5). Osteoporosis is <-2.5. The implication is that the likelihood of fracture (which doubles for each -1 standard deviation) is at least five times normal.

Spinal osteoporosis (porous bones)

Osteoporosis[2] is a very common condition with 1 in 3 women and 1 in 8 men sustaining an osteoporotic-related fracture at some time in their lives. It can be defined *qualitatively* as a reduction in the amount of bone without a change in its composition, with microarchitectural failure, increased fragility and likelihood of fracture; and *quantitatively* as a reduction in bone mass. This is measured as bone mineral density or bone mineral content and is defined as being 2.5 standard deviations or more from the mean peak bone mass. This is expressed as a T score. Osteoporosis arises from an imbalance between bone formation (by osteoblasts) and bone resorption (by osteoclasts) in favour of resorption.

It occurs predominantly in elderly and in post-menopausal women (Table 2) but there are important secondary causes. Osteoporosis particularly affects the trabecular bone in the vertebral bodies which is metabolically more active than cortical bone and changes more quickly in response to alterations in hormones, nutrition and mechanical stimuli.

Table 10.2 The main causes of osteoporosis

Age related	In elderly women and men. Post menopausal
Not related to age (i.e. secondary osteoporosis), e.g. low body mass index, history of anorexia nervosa, smoking, alcohol, drugs – steroids, anticonvulsants; low exercise level, previous fractures.	Oestrogen lack, testosterone lack, corticosteroid excess, malabsorption, coeliac disease, generalized, localized
Endocrine	Osteogenesis imperfecta, Turner's syndrome
Gastrointestinal	
Immobility	In children, in pregnancy
Genetic	Mastocytosis, Satellite travel
Idiopathic	
Rare	

The loss of trabecular bone in osteoporosis makes the vertebrae fragile and leads to compression fractures with minimal trauma. These are typically wedge-shaped. Fractures often but not always cause pain in the back and loss of height. Normally the height of the person is equal to the span, and the distance between crown and pubic symphysis (upper segment) equals that between pubic symphysis to heel (lower segment). In osteoporosis the upper segment height decreases associated with a progressive kyphosis. Spinal cord or root compression does not occur in osteoporotic vertebral collapse and such symptoms should suggest another diagnosis. Loss of height is not always entirely due to osteoporosis and it occurs with ageing due to reduction in the intervertebral disc spaces.

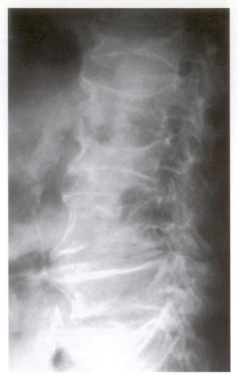

Figure 10.2 Plain X-ray of osteoporotic spine.

Osteoporosis in younger people may produce deformity in the sternum as well as in the spine. The amount of bone in the skeleton depends on peak bone mass (i.e. maximum amount of bone in the young adult) and the rate of subsequent loss. Thus spinal osteoporosis is (in part) prevented by maximizing peak bone mass (exercise, oral calcium, avoiding risk factors) and preventing subsequent loss (by hormone replacement therapy or bisphosphonates where appropriate).

Vertebral fractures due to osteoporosis may occur with little trauma; it is wise to avoid flexion stress on the spine. Although osteoporotic vertebral fracture is said to occur sometimes without pain, pain can be severe, localized and difficult to treat and may take a few weeks to subside. Local support, sufficient analgesics and, according to some, calcitonin injections may be useful. Management of osteoporosis has recently been reviewed in detail.[3]

Paget's disease of bone

Paget's disease is common, particularly amongst the elderly in whom 4–8% are affected worldwide (and about three quarters of a million persons in the UK), especially in Northern industrial towns. The cause is unknown. There is excessive and disorderly activity of bone cells lead by

Table 10.3 Main differential diagnosis of spinal Paget's disease

Disease	Radiology	Main biochemical change*	Comments
Paget's disease	Vertebrae dense, deformed, enlarged	SAP+++	Other bones affected
Metastatic bone disease (osteoblastic secondaries)	Increased density, not enlarged	SAP+, AcP+ if prostate primary	Typically prostatic secondaries
Hyperparathyroidism	Osteoporosis, osteosclerosis, rarely 'cystic'	SAP+, Ca+, P–	Subperiosteal resorption in other areas
Fibrous dysplasia	'Cystic' areas in vertebral bodies	SAP±	Polystotic form exists
Generalized osteosclerosis	Variable appearances	AcP+ in marble bone disease	Myelosclerosis, fluorosis, marble bone disease[6]
Focal osteosclerosis (i.e. one vertebra affected)	Isolated dense vertebra not enlarged		Lymphoma, haemangioma, secondary deposits[4]

*SAP, serum alkaline phosphatase; Ca, P, serum values; AcP, serum acid phosphatase.

the osteoclasts with subsequent deformity, pain and fracture. About 5 per cent of those with Paget's disease have symptoms. The spine is frequently affected. There is enlargement, deformity and collapse of all components of the vertebrae (body, pedicles, neural arches). Isolated vertebrae can be affected. Apart from back pain and loss of height due to vertebral collapse, in contrast to osteoporosis, the most important complication of spinal Paget's disease is compression of the spinal cord and its roots. The extent of this is well demonstrated by CT and MRI scans.

Previous treatment for spinal cord compression due to Paget's disease was surgical; Now modern treatment with bisphosphonates provides a medical alternative. The diagnosis of Paget's disease is based on the clinical findings with deformity and local warmth of the affected bones and a raised plasma alkaline phosphatase, and on the radiological appearances. Occasionally increased density on isolated vertebrae may provide difficulty in diagnosis as may generalized osteosclerosis (Table 3). In pagetic bone there is considerably increased uptake of bone seeking isotope. Very rarely the spine is affected by pagetic sarcoma.

Other bone diseases

Osteomalacia

This is due to lack of vitamin D or a disturbance of its metabolism. There are many causes. The spine is particularly affected in renal glomerular failure and in so called vitamin D-resistant rickets (inherited hypophosphataemia). In the first, there is widespread softening of the skeleton –

including the spine – with vertebral deformity and loss of height. In the second, paraplegia or cord compression can result from ossification of the spinal ligaments (an aspect of the generalized enthesiopathy).

Parathyroid over-activity

This can lead to widespread bone loss with predominant osteoporosis. Very rarely a local brown tumour – osteitis fibrosa cystica – occurs in the vertebrae.

Osteogenesis imperfecta (OI)

OI is a group of disorders due to mutations in the type 1 collagen genes (Type 1 collagen is the major form of collagen in the body and the only type of collagen in bone). The spine is particularly affected in the non-lethal severe form (Type III). Severe progressive kyphoscoliosis occurs. The tissues are in general too fragile for successful operative correction such as spinal fusion.

Chondrodysplasias

This is a large group of rare disorders mainly due to defects in cartilage resulting from mutations in genes of the collagen family. In the spondyloepiphyseal disorders the spine is specifically affected. Neurological complications can arise from an abnormal cervical spine and nerve compression in the thoracolumbar region.

Achondroplasia

This is the commonest form of short-limbed short stature. It is often included amongst the chondrodysplasias but has features of its own. It is inherited as an autosomal dominant disorder. The interpedicular distances in the lower lumbar vertebrae narrow leading to cauda equina compression. Symptoms are most severe where there is an associated thoracolumbar kyphosis. The genetic cause has now been identified.

Marfan's syndrome

This generalized disorder is due to mutations in the gene for fibrillin, a glycoprotein associated with the micro-fibrillar system. The spine may be considerably deformed by a progressive kyphoscoliosis. Tissues such as the aorta and the eyes are affected. The disorder is inherited as a dominant.

Fibrous dysplasia

Often included in the chondrodysplasias, this disorder may affect single (monostotic) or multiple (polyostotic) bones. It is due to a mutation in the G protein signalling system. The expanding cystic appearance in the long bones may closely resemble the resorbing front in Paget's disease. Pain and considerable deformity occur in a polyostotic form; rarely this is associated with pigmentation of the skin and sexual precocity in females (McCune-Albright syndrome).

Alkaptonuria

In this rare disorder due to homogentisic acid oxidase deficiency there is widespread calcification of the intervertebral discs leading to back pain. There is early degenerative arthritis of the major joints. The diagnostic features are dark urine (hence alkaptonuria) and widespread black pigmentation of articular cartilage and elsewhere (hence ochronosis).

Summary

- The main metabolic bone diseases affecting the spine are osteoporosis and Paget's disease.
- Osteoporosis, which is most common in post-menopausal women, leads to bone fragility and vertebral collapse.
- Fracture of the vertebrae causes variable pain, loss of height and eventual kyphosis.
- Prevention of fracture depends on prevention of osteoporosis by sufficient exercise, oral calcium, vitamin D and where appropriate hormone replacement therapy or bisphosphonates.
- Pain in the back, loss of height and vertebral fracture are not always due to osteoporosis, especially in men. Alternative secondary causes of osteoporosis (such as corticosteroid therapy, coeliac disease, thyrotoxicosis) and other diagnoses (metastatic bone disease, myeloma) should be excluded.
- Paget's disease is common and often affects the spine. It may begin in early life; it is progressive and treatable with modern bisphosphonates.
- The bones in Paget's disease become enlarged. This can lead to spinal cord or root compression which requires rapid treatment.
- Many other rare metabolic bone diseases affect the spine. These require specialist advice.

References

1. Smith, R. (1999). Bone in health and disease. In *Oxford Textbook of Rheumatology* (P.J. Maddison, D.A. Isenberg, P. Woo and D.N. Glass, eds) 2nd edn, pp. 421–440, Oxford University Press.
2. Marcus, R., Feldman, D. and Kelsey, J. (1996). *Osteoporosis*. Academic Press.
3. Royal College of Physicians. (1999). *Osteoporosis. Clinical Guidelines for Prevention and Treatment*
4. Kanis, J.A. (1991). *Pathophysiology and Treatment of Paget's Disease of Bone*. Martin Dunitz.
5. Smith, R. and Houghton, G. (1990). Metabolic and inherited disorders of the spine. In *Spinal Surgery Science and Practice* (R.A. Dickson, ed.) pp. 436–482, Butterworths.

Chapter 11

Management of Spinal Deformity in Primary Care

Jeremy Fairbank

Introduction

Spinal deformity is not written large in the pantheon of general practice diagnosis, although school screening studies have detected minor curves in 10 per cent of the adolescent population. Curves sufficient to require specialist observation and treatment are present in 2/1000 adolescent females. Spinal curves are a lot less frequent in boys. The diversity of causes of spinal deformity means that although individually rare in family practice, cumulatively every practice will have several.

This chapter gives a brief overview of the clinical spectrum of spinal deformity, the principles underlying management, and the areas where the GP is likely to be involved in diagnosis or counselling patients through difficult decisions.

Background

This area involves some jargon. Commonly used terms are listed in a glossary. Curves are usually measured by Cobb angle, where 0° is straight and 100° is very bent (curves can be even larger than this). Curves are described by the site and the direction of the convexity. A right thoracic curve is the common pattern in adolescent idiopathic scoliosis. About 80 per cent of new cases of scoliosis are idiopathic in origin. The rest have underlying diagnoses with, in some cases, an obvious reason for the spinal deformity to develop. There is much speculation as to the aetiology of the idiopathic cases. It is likely to involve a combination of minor asymmetries in cerebral function, rapid spinal growth in adolescence and susceptibility of the growth plates to minor asymmetries in loading. It is much more common in girls than boys. About 20 per cent have a family history of the condition.

The engine of curve progression is growth and growth potential. Once skeletal maturity is reached, curve progression is much slower. Larger curves (say greater than 30°) do progress at about 1°/year, as do curves caused by neurological conditions. A curve presenting in a young child has considerable capacity to progress, although some infantile idiopathic curves resolve. The lungs continue to arborize up to the age of 7, so

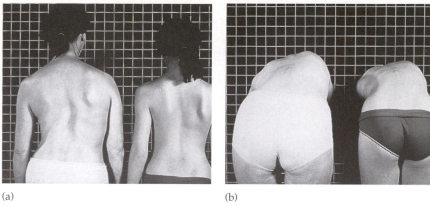

(a)   (b)

Figure 11.1 The forward bending test. Mother and daughter with idiopathic scoliosis. The condition has a family history in up to 20 per cent of cases. No gene has been identified. (a) Standing. (b) Bending forward, hands on knees. [NB this is the best position for seeing a thoracic rib hump. A lumbar curve is best seen with hands on the shins].

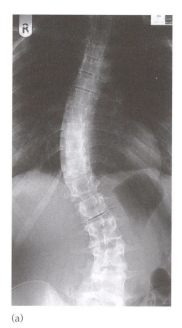

(a)

Figure 11.2 (a) X-ray of a typical thoracic curve of idiopathic scoliosis of about 50°, convex to the right. Note that these films are reversed from the conventional orientation, so as to be seen from behind. (b) The same curve after instrumentation and fusion.

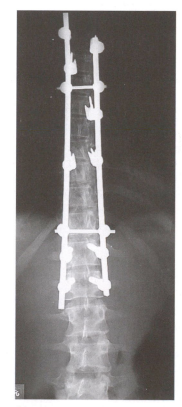

(b)

curves in children younger than this can affect pulmonary function, and ultimately may be life shortening through the later development of cor pulmonale.

The diagnosis depends on someone noticing the curve. To ignore mothers of small babies complaining of spinal deformity is to invite disaster. Adolescents are infrequent attenders in the surgery. They are also less often seen by their parents with their clothes off. Curves are spotted by PE teachers, ballet teachers, school nurses and parents during clothes fittings and summer holidays. Occasionally the patient may notice that clothes do not fit properly or see the rib hump in the mirror. These curves are usually painless, but postural- or fatigue-related back pain can draw attention to the curve. Continuous back pain or night pain is a 'red flag', and must be investigated. Every opportunity should be taken to view the spine in adolescents.

The examination is easy: Ask the subject to bend forward with her hands on her knees and then to touch her toes. Asymmetry of the back is then visible, because rotation of the spine generates a thoracic or lumbar asymmetry (see Fig. 11.1).

A more detailed examination would include an assessment of leg length discrepancy and a neurological examination of the lower limbs.

Investigation is by erect AP and lateral radiographs. This involves significant radiation to a vulnerable age group, and generally I think this is best ordered by the specialist to minimize unnecessary requests (Fig. 11.2).

A 12-year-old girl is brought to your surgery with intermittent thoracic back pain. You examine her spine standing up and bending forward. You note that there is a just detectable asymmetry of the ribcage on the right.

Do you wait and see?
Do you give analgesics and ask the physiotherapist to see her?
Do you send her to the chiropractor?
Ask for urgent paediatric opinion?
Ask for routine orthopaedic opinion?

The orthopaedic surgeon is your best bet. Ideally she should be seen within 3–4 months. If this is not possible, it might be worth seeing her yourself in that time-scale just to make sure that it is not progressing aggressively. If it is, ask for a more urgent appraisal.

Adolescent idiopathic scoliosis

Presents at age 10–15 years in girls, and 12–18 years in boys. The ratio of F:M is 8:1 for large curves, but 1:1 for small curves. The convexity is usually right thoracic (to the point that left thoracic curves are treated with considerable suspicion of an underlying neurological lesion). The scoliosis progresses most rapidly in the peri-menarchal year in girls.

> **The parents of the girl return a year later saying the orthopaedic specialist has done "nothing", and request a second opinion. You re-examine her, and it is obvious that the rib hump is much worse.**
>
> Spine surgeons are used to this, and we are often asked to see patients from elsewhere. There may be good reason for benign neglect, and the parents should have had this explained. However sometimes poor advice has been given, and another surgeon may have a different view.

Management

Observation by radiography or surface topography (optical technology to measure the size of the rib hump) is maintained through growth. If the curve progresses, then it can be treated by benign neglect, exercises, bracing or surgery.

Benign neglect means following the natural history of the condition. The main consequences are 'cosmetic', although these can be quite significant in some individuals. Pain is a feature in some curves, particularly if it involves the lumbar spine, in adults. Whether this is worse than the background incidence of back pain is debatable (see adult scoliosis below). Respiratory function is not usually compromised in the condition. Curves >70° are associated with some loss of vital capacity.

Exercises are widely used, but there is little or no evidence for efficacy. Conflicting advice is given concerning sporting activities. My view is that it is unnecessary to put any restriction on sporting activity. Indeed I would encourage all normal activity. Arguments arise with activities such as horse riding, trampolining, high jumping, parachuting, contact sports etc. There is little evidence for or against these in scoliotics. My view is that so long as the patient has not had surgery, I put no restrictions on their activities. I am not aware that chiropractic treatment can make any difference to the natural history of the condition.

> **The surgeon has recommended a brace. The girl's mother consults you in tears. Her daughter refuses to wear the brace/the school will not let her do PE for fear of harming the girl/family relationships are breaking down/her previously difficult to manage daughter has become impossible.**
>
> Seek local support from practice nurse/community paediatrician/education authorities. Contact the surgeon. Many have experienced physiotherapists involved in bracing clinics who may be able to help. Ultimately the risk/benefits have to be weighed up against the domestic and personal disruption involved. We maintain contact with families that have successfully completed treatment. The Scoliosis Association has an active membership which can provide support.

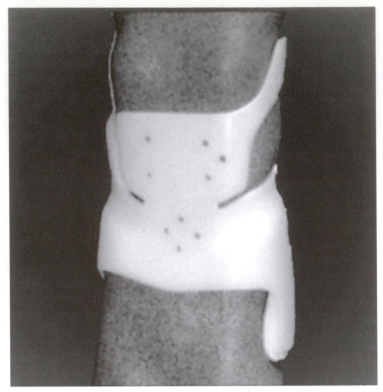

Figure 11.3 Boston Brace (reproduced with kind permission from the Boston Brace Company, Avon, Massachusetts, USA).

Bracing is used to prevent progression in growth. The evidence for this is hotly debated. Bracing is an unpleasant experience at a vulnerable time in development, and can cause considerable family stress and guilt. This needs sympathetic handling by all concerned, and an open discussion of the management decisions. Braces are supposed to be worn 23 hours/ day, but may be removed for sport and exercise. A detailed account of the 'anti-bracing' position can be found in a recent editorial.[1] A Boston Brace is illustrated in Fig. 11.3.

> **The parents come to see you to say that the surgeon has offered surgery. Their daughter wishes to proceed, but the parents are scared by the long list of risks presented to them by the surgeon.**
>
> There is usually no rush about making a decision. Surgeons are used to families returning several times before making up their minds. Some provide counselling by hospital nurses or physiotherapists. Other will put families in contact with others who have had surgery. Sometimes a second opinion is helpful.

Surgery is used to correct and stabilize the larger curves (>40°). Fifty per cent or greater correction of the Cobb angle is usually possible, but the rib hump may persist (unless reduced by direct rib excision – a costoplasty) or recur if the child still has growth potential. The main objective is to improve cosmesis and prevent progression. If pain is present, surgery usually relieves it. Spine surgery of all sorts carries high risks of litigation, and you should find that the specialist has been frank and clear over the risks of surgery. If your patient has not been made aware of or does not seem to understand the risks, this should be pointed out to the surgeon. We tell patients that there is a 1 per cent risk of spinal cord damage up to and including complete paraplegia (the term should be explained as unable to walk, wheelchair-dependent, with loss of micturition, bowel and sexual functions). There is up to a 10 per cent risk of repeat surgery to remove implants for pain, infection, loosening, pseudarthrosis and implant failure. Some surgeons use postoperative bracing. Adolescents should be able to return to school from about 4 weeks post-surgery. Return to normal activities depends on the procedure, surgeon and patient. I usually allow swimming from 3 months, and all but the most violent sport from 6 months post-surgery. In the longer term, on somewhat irrational grounds, I discourage sports involving falls from heights.

Surgical treatment involves tough decisions for all concerned. The ultimate decision is usually taken by the child herself. Solace may be taken from the maturity that is often shown by our patients and (sometimes) their parents. Those interested in this area may benefit from studying Patricia Alderson's work.[2]

The parents of a 10-year-old child with cerebral palsy present. This is a much-loved member of the family who has had the full resources of the local paediatric services available to him. Recently he has had major readjustment to his seating because of increasing pelvic obliquity. The orthopaedic surgeon has recommended a major anterior and posterior correction of the spine to correct some of the deformity and prevent progression. He has explained that there are serious risks attached to the surgery including a small risk to life. The parents have seen another child in their son's special school who has had surgery that has been successful.

This is a very difficult decision for parents who often carry a lot of guilt. They are very distressed by taking a decision for their son that he cannot partake in. All parties can help here. Again there is not too much rush about the decision. Some doctors are unhappy about devoting precious resources to children in these circumstances at the expense of other more able patients. The long-term consequences of non-stabilization are serious, and can make it very difficult to care for these children. See a recent paper from Japan on the natural history of these children.[3]

Neuromuscular (paralytic) scoliosis

Neuromuscular is used in a wider sense than used by neurologists to include all neurological disorders affecting children. Table 11.1 has a list of the more common categories in this very long list of conditions. In the past poliomyelitis was by far the commonest reason for spinal deformity, and the polio era generated many of the techniques we use today. Fortunately polio is largely behind us, to be replaced by cerebral palsy as the main diagnosis in this group. Sadly, although modern obstetric and neonatal practice has had many benefits, there are still many children with cerebral palsy. In essence the more severe the involvement, particularly if the child cannot stand or walk, the more likely is spinal deformity to develop. Most of these children are managed by community paediatric services and physiotherapists. Difficult decisions need to be taken about the appropriateness and timing of surgery. Practice varies considerably from one centre to another.

Table 11.1 Conditions associated with neuromuscular scoliosis (incomplete list)

Cerebral palsy
Myelodysplasia (spinal dysraphism)
Rett's syndrome
Poliomyelitis
Muscular dystrophies, especially Duchenne muscular dystrophy
Syringomyelia (commonly associated with congenital scoliosis)
Familial dysautonomia (Riley-Day)
Malignant hyperpyrexia

Duchenne muscular dystrophy is often associated with scoliosis once the boy goes off his feet at around the age of 10–11 years. Surgery has a place in preventing progression of deformity and its adverse effect on respiratory function.

> **A mother of an 8-month-old boy keeps bringing him to the surgery complaining that his spine is bent. The spine looked straight to your partner who saw him last time. It looks pretty normal to you, but he does have a small hairy patch in the midline at about the level of L2.**
>
> There is no substitute for an X-ray here. Probably this is best initiated by an orthopaedic surgeon or a paediatrican. If there is spinal deformity, then he will be referred on to the orthopaedic surgeon in any case. A neurosurgeon may also be involved if there are cord anomalies or an Arnold-Chiari malformation.

Congenital scoliosis

This represents about 5 per cent of specialist practice. There is failure of formation of segmentation of the spine. Deformity ranges from the trivial to the horrendous. These are mesenchymal and ectodermal development failures which are usually non-genetic. They are frequently associated with cardiac and urogenital abnormalities, and there may be abnormalities of the spinal cord and brainstem (syrinx, split cords, tethered cords, diastematomyelia and Arnold-Chiari malformations). Many are

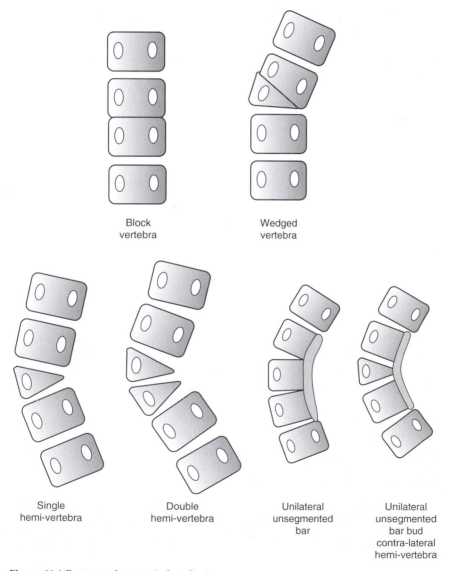

Block
vertebra

Wedged
vertebra

Single
hemi-vertebra

Double
hemi-vertebra

Unilateral
unsegmented
bar

Unilateral
unsegmented
bar bud
contra-lateral
hemi-vertebra

Figure 11.4 Patterns of congenital scoliosis.

diagnosed from routine postnatal chest X-rays taken in neonates with cardiopulmonary conditions. An increasing number are identified on antenatal ultrasound. The rest present with deformity usually noticed by their mothers. Sometimes there are midline hairy patches, dimples etc. over the spine. Foot deformities and leg length discrepancies are common. They tend to be shorter than expected from parental heights. Figure 11.4 illustrates some of the many patterns of malformation.

Management depends on the potential for progression that is estimated from asymmetry of growth plates. The most malignant pattern is where there are no growth plates on one side and three or more on the other (the 'unsegmented bar'). If caught early enough, it can be treated with a growth arrest procedure (epiphyseodesis) on the front and the back of the spine. Bracing is usually pretty hopeless, but can be helpful for less threatening patterns. Corrective surgery by osteotomy or instrumentation is possible, but the usual risks of paraplegia are increased by the presence of spinal cord anomalies. The widening availability of MRI means that this investigation is now essential before surgery is attempted. Foramen magnum decompression may be indicated for Arnold-Chiari malformations.

The 10-year-old daughter of a large family in your practice presents with a small rib hump. She is known to have neurofibromatosis (type 1), of which most are only mildly affected.

There is debate about the level of cover that should be offered to families with NF1.[4] This child should be reviewed by an orthopaedic surgeon.

Syndromal scoliosis

There are many syndromes of children that may include scoliosis. A less than exhaustive list of the more frequent conditions are given in Table 11.2. Neurofibromatosis Type 1 (von Recklinghausen's disease) is the commonest (1:5000). Spinal deformities occur in about 10–20% and are particularly troublesome to treat because of a high pseudarthrosis rate following fusion and because of associated involvement of the spine and spinal cord. Otherwise these scolioses are managed according to the general principles articulated above.

Table 11.2 Syndromal scoliosis – the more common causes

Neurofibromatosis (Type 1)
Inherited connective tissue disorders (esp osteogenisis imperfecta; Marfan's)
Mucopolysaccharidoses
Bone dysplasias
Metabolic bone disease

> **A 15-year-old boy presents with his mother because of a bilateral rib hump. He has no pain. The hump does not look too bad to you.**
>
> An X-ray of the spine is helpful here (erect is best). If it is reported as normal, observe. If he has Scheuermann's disease, it is probably best to refer as routine.

Idiopathic kyphosis (Scheuermann's disease)

Scheuermann's disease affects boy and girls, with, probably, a male predominance. It is a radiological diagnosis of altered growth plates, vertebral body wedging and Schmorl's nodes (disc herniations through the endplate). It is frequently asymptomatic, but may be associated with back pain, which usually resolves at skeletal maturity. Others get a kyphosis that may be of considerable cosmetic consequence (in an extreme example, I recently saw an otherwise normal teenage boy who would not go out of the house because of his appearance. Surgery has cured this problem). The long-term effects of a Scheuermann's kyphosis is otherwise benign. This curve will respond to bracing. Surgery is only considered for large curves (say >80°, the normal range being 20–40°). It involves an anterior release via thoracotomy followed by posterior instrumentation and fusion. This is major surgery with a definite risk of cord damage. The correction obtainable is unpredictable, and sometimes disappointing. Spine surgeons are therefore unenthusiastic about this type of surgery.

Other causes of kyphosis

Angular kyphoses secondary to congenital hemivertebrae, tuberculosis, and occasionally fracture tend to progress, even after skeletal maturity, and will cause spinal cord compression. In general spinal cord compression due to kyphosis requires anterior decompression and stabilization. Some cases require posterior fusion as well. Kyphosis correction carries a significant risk to spinal cord function.

> **A 51-year-old woman has complained intermittently of back pain for years. She attends for the first time for a year, saying it has got worse, and she can only walk for 200 metres before she has to sit down. You examine her, and are surprised to find a lumbar hump in the left. She tells you it has gradually appeared over the last year.**
>
> This probably needs a specialist opinion, but it is worth trying usual non-operative measures such as analgesics and physiotherapy. Corsets may be helpful, although their use has declined considerably.

Adults with spinal deformity

The majority of these date from childhood. Often they will have been told at skeletal maturity that their deformity would not progress. They are upset and angry when it does. Surgical horizons have expanded considerably in the last 20 years, and surgery is now done on adult deformity, certainly up the age of 50. However there are more complications than there are in the teenagers. This provides some argument for doing the surgery in teenagers, especially as they do not (usually) have dependants. Some adults are deeply upset by their appearances, and may be resentful of their parents if they were 'stopped' from having surgery. They may also be upset if they spent many years in a brace, only to be told they need an operation, which is what the brace was supposed to be preventing. The main reason that adults opt for surgery is when there is uncontrolled pain.

There are a group of adults presenting with *de novo* scoliosis (degenerative scoliosis). This affects particularly the lumbar spine and is very difficult to manage. Pain is often distressing, though usually relieved by rest. Some have neurogenic claudication. Non-operative means include corsets, traction and physiotherapy. Surgery is difficult and carries a high complication rate. Our audits suggest the complication rate becomes unacceptable over the age of 60. Sometimes we can get away with nerve root surgery to relieve claudication without destabilizing the whole spine.

A previously fit 75-year-old female presents with increasing kyphosis. She developed back pain acutely a week ago. Direct questioning reveals a recent history of weight loss.

This is likely to be an osteoporotic collapse, and can be diagnosed by X-ray. If the pain continues or deteriorates, consider malignancy. ESR/viscosity, CRP, Ca and alkaline phosphatase levels may be abnormal.

Adult kyphosis usually relates to osteoporotic collapse. This should be managed symptomatically. Transcutaneous nerve stimulation may be helpful if collapse is painful, but often it is not. Surgery is rarely indicated, and carries high complication rates. Anyone over the age of 60 (some guidelines say 55) with persisting back pain, night pain or rest pain may have a malignancy. MRI is the best way of diagnosing it, but it is not easy to judge who should get it when resources are limited. If the pattern of pain or symptoms are out of the ordinary, then you should be on alert for this diagnosis.

This is a difficult area, and I believe that it is quite reasonable to refer to specialist for discussion of the issues – something some GP's prefer to avoid for fear of wasting resources.

Summary

- Take every opportunity of performing a forward bend test on adolescents.
- Ignore mothers of small babies complaining of spinal deformities at your peril.
- Refer all children and adolescents in whom any suspicion of spinal deformity.

References

1. Dickson, R.A. (1999). Spinal deformity – adolescent idiopathic scoliosis. Nonoperative treatment. *Spine*, **24**, 2601–2606.
2. Alderson, P. (1993). Children's consent to treatment. Abstract debate is unhelpful. *BMJ*, **307**(6898), 260–261.
3. Saito, N., Ebara, S., Ohotsuka, H., Kumeta, H. and Takaoka, K. (1998). Natural history of scoliosis in spastic cerebral palsy. *Lancet*, **351**:1687–1692.
4. Huson, S.M. (1999). What level of care for the neurofibromatoses? *Lancet*, **353**(9159), 1114–1116.

Investigations

Chapter 12

Radiological Investigation and Management of Lumbosacral Pain

Paul O'Donnell and Eugene McNally

Introduction

Management and investigation of low back pain (LBP) in primary care is such a difficult subject that it is almost impossible to give a didactic account in one short chapter. There are clear guidelines from the Royal Colleges of General Practitioners and Radiologists on which group of patients should be investigated, in order to separate sinister causes of low back pain from benign. However, clinical presentation is often non-specific and some patients with serious underlying pathology may not be adequately investigated despite the clinician remaining within the guidelines.

The problem

The problem with respect to imaging is one of correlating clinical symptoms and radiological findings. Degenerative changes are ubiquitous, obviously increasing with patient age. There may be multiple abnormalities on imaging, any one of which may be responsible for symptoms. For example, X-ray computed tomography (CT) and magnetic resonance imaging (MRI) elegantly demonstrate facet joint osteoarthritis, but the appearances do not correlate with severity of symptoms: intra-articular injection of local anaesthetic if it relieves the symptoms, may be regarded as a moderate measure of demonstrating the joint responsible for symptoms.

Similar problems are encountered with discogenic pain and nerve root compression in patients with spondylosis – the initial imaging tests show lesions, but the significance of these abnormalities needs confirmation by other means.

Pain with radiation into the legs is a common diagnostic challenge with multiple causes. Distinction of true nerve root pain from other conditions where pain may be referred is often difficult.

There are a large number of potential investigations available, even once the difficult decision of who to investigate has been made. The investigations have differing sensitivities, and are appropriate for different pathologies. The correct selection is, principally, based on clinical assessment, which may be confusing. The investigation of patients will, unfortunately, be partly determined by local availability, waiting lists and financial considerations.

Aims

Radiological investigation should be aimed at determining the cause of back symptoms for management purposes. It should detect surgical lesions, giving detail on both appropriate level and operative approach. It should also prevent the surgeon from operating inappropriately or at the wrong level, the latter being a major cause of failed back surgery. If the patient is not a surgical candidate or with non-surgical lesions, imaging will exclude sinister, non-mechanical causes of symptoms, and direct patients away from surgery to more appropriate conservative treatments. Symptoms may already have suggested the correct diagnosis, with radiology simply being used to exclude more sinister pathology.

Provocative or anaesthetic procedures are also useful in the diagnosis of the source of pain. Some interventions, for example discography (see below), which invariably follow cross-sectional imaging, should be restricted to patients who are being considered for surgery. Patients may occasionally obtain prolonged relief from local anaesthetic injections, which may therefore be used therapeutically as well as diagnostically. More permanent therapies can also be performed percutaneously in selected patients, for example treatment of facet joint pain, although the evidence to support this approach is not robust.

In the presence of radicular or stenotic symptoms (back pain with neural pain), radiological investigation determines the level and nature of the compressive lesion. With equivocal cases, further tests can assess the significance of any impingement before the patient is subjected to surgery. In other cases of referred pain from the back, which may simulate true nerve root pain, imaging can exclude compression of a nerve root.

Surgical candidates with nerve root pain may be treated percutaneously as well as surgically.

Techniques

Plain radiographs of lumbosacral spine

Only a small proportion of the patients presenting with LBP requires investigation. Not only is the plain radiograph insensitive, and unable to detect significant pathologies, it may also be falsely reassuring, showing normal appearances at symptomatic levels. If MRI is available, there is no indication for performing plain X-rays.

The standard plain radiographic assessment of the lumbar spine consists of anteroposterior and lateral views. Some information on the distribution of bony degenerative changes, loss of disc height and presence of spinal stenosis can be obtained, in addition to the presence of bone destruction. Patients with a degree of spinal instability often have a suggestive history – plain films may show malalignment and traction spur formation in keeping with the diagnosis.

However, this investigation is insensitive even to the conditions for which it is indicated. Plain film demonstration of spondylotic changes is of little clinical benefit, as it will generally not assist patient management. Disc degenerative changes (loss of height, end plate sclerosis, and osteophyte formation) correlate poorly with discogenic pain or instability – symptoms may equally be originating at another, apparently preserved disc or another source entirely.

In younger patients (less than 30 years), demonstration of degeneration at a single disc level may be more significant. Radiographs show facet joint osteoarthritis only moderately, and are unable to show soft tissue abnormalities that are often responsible for symptoms. Facet joint changes may be demonstrated by other techniques but no correlation between the clinical and radiological features is consistently demonstrated.[1]

Plain X-rays are insensitive to marrow infiltration and early bone destruction, and therefore gives only limited exclusion of sinister causes of backache. The posterior elements, a common site for metastases, are often not well demonstrated. Finally, X-rays of the lumbosacral spine involve the largest dose of radiation to the patient from any plain radiographic study, equivalent to approximately 7 months of background radiation exposure, which, in view of its limitations, is usually unjustified, unless no other imaging technique is available.

X-ray computed tomography (CT)

Axial imaging using CT gives the best morphologic detail of bony structures of all the available imaging techniques. It was previously the

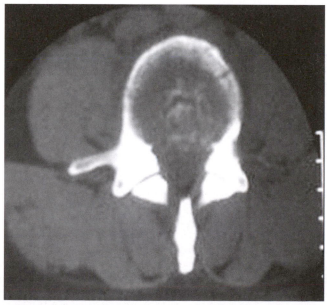

Figure 12.1 CT scan of lumbar vertebra showing pathological fracture secondary to metastases (the primary is bronchial carcinoma). With permission from the South Bank University, London.

investigation of choice for disc prolapse. It is, however, unable to demonstrate the entire spine without unacceptable radiation dose, and cannot therefore be used as a screening examination in patients with low back pain.

CT has a complementary role as a problem-solving device after MRI or plain radiographs have detected a lesion. MRI commonly identifies focal bone lesions incidentally, and CT is required in some of these cases to assess the degree of bone destruction and other potentially aggressive features. Plain films are insensitive to the presence of pars defects and CT can confirm integrity of the bone of the pars intra-articularis. CT is still indicated in the investigation of disc prolapse in patients with nerve root pain and contraindications to MRI.

Magnetic resonance imaging (MRI)

The advantages of MRI are now well known. Without the use of ionizing radiation, large segments of the spine can be imaged quickly and accurately. Imaging in the three standard orthogonal planes (axial, sagittal and coronal), and obliquely, adds a further advantage over CT. Sagittal and axial images generally suffice for demonstration of the lumbar spine. However the greatest advantage of MRI is the increased sensitivity to soft tissue pathology, as it provides much better soft tissue contrast when compared with CT. The use of multiple sequences further increases the sensitivity of the examination. Its disadvantage is that it detects something 'abnormal' in everyone, and these abnormalities are not always clinically significant.

A number of techniques are available to suppress the high signal returned by fat, resulting in pathology becoming more prominent. Early oedema associated with degenerative, inflammatory and malignant lesions can therefore be appreciated long before plain films become abnormal. The paramagnetic contrast agent gadolinium can also be administered intravenously, but due to the sensitivity of MRI to soft tissue pathology, is perhaps less of a routine addition to standard investigations than use of iodinated contrast media in CT.

Investigation of the lumbar spine is probably the most common indication for MRI. In nerve root pain, it can demonstrate the site and cause of nerve root impingement. Unilateral symptoms are commonly due to either a disc protrusion, or stenosis of either the nerve root exit foramen or lateral recess, which may be multifactorial: these patients often have diffuse spondylotic changes, and there may be more than one possible source of symptoms. In nerve root pain due to disc protrusion, MRI shows the level of the affected disc, the position of disc material and the suitability of the lesion to percutaneous treatment. Occasionally, there are multiple disc protrusions and, again, it may not be possible definitively to identify the symptomatic lesion. The side of symptoms is perhaps the most important clinical detail that needs to be included on the request card; without this, an assessment of the most likely cause is often not possible. Supplementary nerve root block with local anaesthetic, when positive, will confirm the affected root. It is important to emphasize that an appearance of nerve root compression does not always correlate with symptoms.

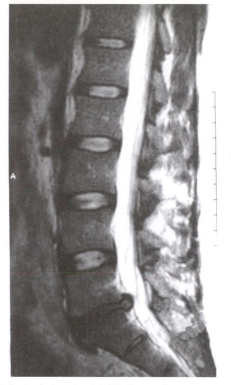

Figure 12.2 MRI (sagittal view) showing L5/S1 disc prolapse.

Contraindications to MRI

Absolute contraindications are:

Pacemakers
Intracranial metal work especially aneurysm clips
Certain types of cardiac valve replacements*
Certain types of endovascular prostheses*
Cochlear implants
Intra-orbital metal fragments

Relative contra-indications are:

Pregnancy especially first trimester. MR possible in life threatening circumstances

*Not all endovascular and valve implants are contraindicated and specific advice should be sought in each case. Your local MR unit will have a list of MR-incompatible devices.

If symptoms are bilateral, spinal stenosis affecting exit foramina, lateral recesses or central canal may be present. There are normally multiple contributory factors to central canal stenosis, but there is generally an underlying congenitally narrow spinal canal that, with additional degenerative hypertrophy of ligaments and facet joints, becomes symptomatic.[2] Myelography was previously the investigation of choice, and is still used if MRI is contraindicated or if there has been metallic spinal fixation. Stenosis affecting the lateral recesses is also normally a degenerative phenomenon involving disc and facet OA. Patients with central or lateral recess stenosis may give the history of pain precipitated or aggravated by walking (spinal extension), and relieved by sitting or squatting. MRI can identify the level that requires decompression, and the cause of the stenosis, with greater accuracy than plain films.

In patients suffering from back pain without leg pain, MRI has a number of advantages over plain radiographs. It gives a more comprehensive overview of degenerative changes, is able to assess areas of the spine poorly shown by plain films, and, perhaps most importantly, is more sensitive to focal bone lesions and marrow infiltration.

Degenerative changes

The internal structure of the intervertebral disc, consisting of a high signal nucleus pulposus and a peripheral, low signal annulus fibrosus, is best demonstrated by MR images with T2 weighting. Loss of nuclear signal, often accompanied by subtle loss of disc height, is one of the earliest signs of degeneration detectable by MRI, and may be radiographically occult. This process can even start in teenagers. Although it is often asymptomatic, disc degeneration is related to low back pain in a significant proportion of those scanned. The precise proportion is unknown.

There may be accompanying annular changes, from degenerative bulging of the annulus around the entire circumference of the disc, to small peripheral fissures within the annulus. These appear as focal areas of increased signal within the normally homogeneously black periphery of the disc, and are thought by some authors to be closely correlated with a painful disc.[3]

Facet arthropathy may be a contributing cause of simple back pain and changes can be detected on both axial and sagittal images. The usual imaging features of OA, including cartilage loss, joint effusions, osteophyte and synovial cyst formation, can all be demonstrated. As symptoms are often out of proportion to the appearances of the joint, the diagnosis of facet joint pain is occasionally one of exclusion. Ghormley first postulated the concept of facet joints as a source of pain with typical radiation in 1933.[4] Subsequent authors have shown that injection of hypertonic saline into the joints of normal volunteers causes local pain and referred pain into the ipsilateral buttock and thigh.[5]

There are no diagnostic clinical or radiological appearances, but the presence of back pain with typical referred pain to the groin or thigh, paraspinal tenderness, reproduction of symptoms with extension-rotation movements, and significant radiological abnormalities, may be consistent with the so-called facet joint syndrome.[6] The facet joint can be confirmed as the source of pain by injection of local anaesthetic, either directly into the joint, or around the medial branch of the lumbar dorsal ramus which supplies the joint. Synovial cysts arising from degenerate facet joints are sometimes associated with pressure on a nerve root within the lateral recess of the spinal canal, causing nerve root pain. Facet joint injection with steroid leads to resolution of these cysts in a proportion of cases.[7]

Areas poorly shown by X-ray

Sagittal MRI sections with a slice thickness of 4 mm or less are able to assess the pars intra-articularis. Standard plain films cannot exclude pars defects (spondylolysis), and special oblique views are required for complete exclusion of a defect. Pars defects are rarely clinically suspected unless associated with marked spondylolisthesis. At the level of the slip, there is invariably disc degeneration and exit foraminal narrowing, and so the cause of the pain may not be entirely clear. Local anaesthetic block of the pars defect itself can isolate this as a source of pain. Spondylolisthesis due to pars defects is more likely to affect adolescents and young adults – degenerative slips are found in older patients with advanced facet OA and subluxation, but intact pars. Similarly, MRI is more sensitive to posterior element pathology than plain films. Again, many patients have these changes without symptoms.

Increased sensitivity to marrow lesions

Non-mechanical causes of LBP are also detected more sensitively using MRI. Early marrow infiltration, before the development of overt bone destruction, may not be appreciated on plain radiographs. MRI is sensitive to any condition that leads to replacement of fatty vertebral marrow, especially if associated with oedema. Thus, diffuse infiltration (as in lymphoma, leukaemia or myeloma) or multiple focal abnormalities (multiple malignant or benign tumours) are sensitively detected. Metastases without marked surrounding oedema may be extremely subtle, but should be detected if more than one sequence is employed.

MRI is such a sensitive technique that benign incidental findings are common. Vertebral body haemangiomata, for example, are frequently seen. They only cause symptoms when aggressive or large, leading to vertebral body collapse. Although plain films are fairly accurate in the diagnosis of vertebral collapse due to osteoporosis, and the absence of detectable bone destruction is reassuring, MRI gives greater exclusion of malignancy as a cause of the collapse. It increases the certainty that there is no paravertebral soft tissue mass, and can also age the fracture, depending on the amount of oedema present. Normal marrow signal returns to chronic wedge fractures,[8] and the appearances tend to be non-progressive. It also detects osteoporotic fractures before there has been significant collapse, which are potential causes of symptoms that would be occult radiographically.

Inflammatory back pain, including spinal infection and spondyloarthritis can be diagnosed earlier on MRI than on plain films. Infective discitis is staged accurately by MRI, which not only shows the degree of bone destruction visible on X-ray, but also shows the extent of vertebral infection, the size and position of the paravertebral abscess and the encroachment on the spinal canal by inflammatory tissue. In ankylosing spondylitis, pre-erosive oedema can be seen at the vertebral corners, reflecting early enthesitis, and also at the costovertebral articulations.

Further investigations and therapeutic procedures

Facet joint

Imaging is unable to demonstrate that a facet joint is the source of pain – pain may still originate from a joint that appears normal. Diagnostic procedures to identify the painful level are possible and are usually performed following exclusion of more serious pathology by MRI, and in patients with a suggestive history. Local anaesthetic blocks at sequential levels may be required. Benefit may be prolonged if steroid is also injected, adding a therapeutic dimension to the technique, but benefit rarely lasts for more than 3 months.[9] If pain is shown to be originating in a facet joint, percutaneous methods aimed at permanent denervation, so called rhizolysis, can be attempted. A number of papers have suggested that the results of facet joint blocks cannot predict surgical outcome,[10] and even questioned the existence of a 'facet syndrome'.[11]

Intra-articular lumbar facet joint blocks
Intra-articular injection of long-acting local anaesthetic and steroid, using fluoroscopic guidance. Position of needle may be confirmed with injection of iodinated contrast media. These are performed with patient prone.

Lumbar medial branch blocks
Local anaesthetic blockade of the medial branch of the lumbar dorsal ramus, which innervates the facet joint, as it crosses the root of the transverse process. These are performed with patient prone, under fluoroscopic control.

Nerve root

Imaging is successful at diagnosing definite nerve root compression, but ancillary tests are occasionally required if findings are equivocal or if more than one nerve root may be responsible for symptoms. The clinical significance of neural impingement and the nerve root responsible for nerve root pain can be elucidated by anaesthetizing the nerve root, referred to as a root block. Equivocal findings on MRI include partial nerve root compression or abutment without displacement, and early foraminal or lateral recess narrowing. Prolonged benefit from this procedure is rare, as the short-acting local anaesthetic agent lignocaine is generally used to avoid motor weakness. The technique is generally restricted to patients being considered for surgery.

Lumbar nerve root blocks
Local anaesthetic block of the lumbar root as it exits from the foramen, inferior to the pedicle. These are performed with patient prone, under fluoroscopic control.

Discography

MRI can identify disc degeneration but is unable to confirm that a disc is painful. When conservative management has failed and surgical fusion is contemplated, provocation of degenerate discs should confirm which one is the source of pain. The aim is to reproduce the patient's usual symptoms by injection of iodinated contrast media directly into a disc. Normal discs are not painful; injection in abnormal discs may provoke pain that is identical or dissimilar, and its assessment is therefore crucial, as fusion is only indicated if the source of pain is confirmed. Some information on the morphology of the disc is obtained, but this may not be diagnostically useful – pain rarely originates from discs that are normal on MRI. Sometimes multiple levels are involved, which may preclude surgical treatment. Discography will also confirm normality in adjacent discs, thereby determining the extent of fusion. It is also helpful in assessing patients with inappropriate responses to pain.

Discography
Injection of contrast into the disc in order to provoke familiar discogenic pain in patients considered for spinal fusion. These are performed with patient lateral under fluoroscopic control, with sedation and antibiotic prophylaxis to avoid disc infection.

Percutaneous therapy

Disc

Percutaneous management of disc prolapse is indicated in a proportion of patients who are suitable for surgery. In patients with nerve root pain, percutaneous treatment avoids the risks of back surgery, but does not prevent its future use. Not all disc lesions are suitable, i.e. those that have a breached annulus as opposed to those with an intact annulus, but this technique is successful in appropriate patients (up to 75 per cent success at 10 years[12]).

Chemonucleolysis using chymopapain, a proteolytic enzyme extracted from the papaya is the most frequently used percutaneous treatment in Oxford. Alternatives are laser discectomy and percutaneous nucleotomy. Complications include 1 per cent risk of discitis and less than 1 per cent risk of anaphylaxes.

Facet
Patients with proven facet joint pain (that is, consistently positive responses to facet injection or medial branch block) can be treated percutaneously by radiofrequency ablation of the medial branch of the lumbar dorsal ramus. The nerve can be destroyed by means of an

electrode introduced down a fine needle placed adjacent to the nerve.[13] If symptoms recur, facet joint fusion may be required.

Vertebra
A number of lesions can be responsible for vertebral collapse, with or without pain. These include benign and malignant tumours, osteoporosis and infection. Percutaneous insertion of methyl methacrylate cement can prevent further collapse and provide a degree of mechanical stabilization, thereby relieving pain. The commonest indications for percutaneous vertebroplasty are palliative treatment for secondary tumours, osteoporotic fractures with prolonged disabling symptoms despite medical treatment and haemangiomas accompanied by severe pain or aggressive radiological features.

Suggested algorithm for radiological investigation of lumbar pain
The limited lumbar spine MRI
Lumbar spine MRI is more sensitive than routine plain X-ray, but time consuming and relatively expensive. The time required for each examination is halved if axial images are not performed, and these can be safely omitted if there is no dominant leg pain. Occasionally there is an incidental finding which necessitates recall for axial imaging. The remaining sagittal sequences provide a comprehensive screening study of the lumbosacral and lower thoracic spines, accurately excluding infection, spinal tumour, acute or chronic vertebral collapse and pars defects. Pre-erosive changes of inflammatory back pain will be detected prior to plain film changes. If none of these lesions is seen, disc and facet pathology will be more completely shown, and an alternative, less sinister cause of pain may be suggested.

In the enviable setting of a dedicated orthopaedic hospital, it has been possible for us to abandon lumbar spine radiographs in the routine investigation of lumbar pain. The clinical information provided on the request form determines whether a limited study is appropriate: it should not be used to investigate the cause of suspected nerve root pain or neurogenic claudication. Thus, if lumbar spine plain films are requested, a limited MRI will invariably be performed.

Cost of limited MRI

A limited MR scan is approximately 50 per cent more than conventional lumbar spine X-ray series and 50 per cent less than a full MRI.

Imaging is not routinely indicated in simple back pain. If atypical features exist, suggesting that investigation is desirable, then we believe that a limited MRI is appropriate, assuming that there are no radiating symptoms.

Patients whose main symptom is leg pain should not undergo a limited MRI. If conservative management has failed, or if therapeutic intervention is planned, a full lumbar spine MRI including axial images at the appropriate level should be considered. MRI should be performed as an emergency in patients with acute cauda equina symptoms and signs.

If a single disc protrusion is identified, which is compatible with the patient's symptoms and signs, and surgery is contemplated, percutaneous treatment may be appropriate by clinical and imaging criteria. If a single equivocal lesion is identified, without definite root compression, or if there are multiple possible lesions, nerve root blocks can be used to assess the symptoms attributable to each level, and to direct surgical decompression.

Conclusion

Despite the presence of guidelines,[14] the decision on whom to investigate will always be difficult. Investigation of patients with simple back pain is often unrewarding. They will invariably have a range of degenerative changes, which, by using second-line tests, may be shown to be relevant. There may be unexpected findings in a small proportion. The purpose of investigation is to find a treatable lesion and exclude a non-mechanical cause – in this regard, a limited MRI scan gives the best exclusion of sinister pathology, and most appropriate triage. In the presence of nerve root pain, MRI is the best test to demonstrate the cause and suitability for percutaneous treatment.

References

1. Bogduk, N., Aprill, C. and Derby, R. (1995). Lumbar zygapophyseal joint pain: diagnostic blocks and therapy. In *Interventional Radiology of the Musculoskeletal System* (D.J. Wilson, ed.) pp. 74–75, Edward Arnold.
2. Resnick, D. (1996). Degenerative disease of the spine. In *Bone and Joint Imaging* (D. Resnick, ed.) pp. 374, W.B. Saunders.
3. Colhoun, E., McCall, I., Williams, W. and Cassar-Pullicino, V. (1988). Provocative discography as a guide to planning operations on the spine. *J. Bone Joint Surg.*, **70B**, 267–271.
4. Ghormley, R. (1933). Low back pain with special reference to the articular facets with presentation of an operative procedure. *JAMA*, **101**, 1773.
5. McCall, I., Park, W. and O'Brien, P. (1979). Induced pain referral from the posterior lumbar elements in normal subjects. *Spine*, **4**, 441–446.
6. Helbig, T. and Lee, C. (1988). The lumbar facet syndrome. *Spine*, **13**, 61–64.
7. Bjorkengren, A., Kurz, L., Resnick, D., Sartoris, D. and Garfin, S. (1987). Symptomatic intraspinal synovial cysts: opacification and treatment by percutaneous injection. *Am. J. Roentgenol.*, **149**(1), 105–107.
8. Yuh, W., Zachar, C., Barloon, T. *et al.* (1989). Vertebral compression fractures: distinction between benign and malignant causes with MR imaging. *Radiology*, **172**, 215–218.
9. Marks, R., Hampton, T. and Thulbourne, T. (1992). Facet joint injection and facet nerve block: a randomised comparison in 86 patients with chronic low back pain. *Pain*, **49**(3), 325–328.

10. Esses, S. and Moro, J. (1993). Value of facet joint injection in selection for lumbar fusion. *Spine*, **18**(2), 185–190.

11. Jackson, R. (1992). The facet syndrome. Myth or reality? *Clin. Orthop. Rel. Res.*, **279**, 110–121.

12. Gogan, W. and Fraser, R. (1992). Chymopapain: a 10-year double-blind study. *Spine*, **17**, 388–394.

13. Yamagami, H., Hashizume, K., Nakahashi, K. and Okuda, T. (1990). Percutaneous radiofrequency neurotomy of lumbar medial branch (facet rhizotomy) – a report of 6 cases. *Jap. J. Anesthesiol.*, **39**(4), 491–495.

14. The Royal College of Radiologists. (1998). *Making the Best Use of a Department of Clinical Radiology: Guidelines for Doctors*. Fourth edition.

Chapter 13

Laboratory Investigations for Low Back Pain

Daniel Porter

Introduction

The early diagnosis of suspected serious pathology will have a major impact on outcome, and laboratory tests are a critical adjunct to history and examination in discrimination of mechanical from non-mechanical causes of back pain. History and examination are the most useful tools for evaluation of low back pain, but it is often difficult for the primary healthcare professional to discriminate between mechanical and non-mechanical aetiologies early in the disease process, since nociceptive stimuli from both utilize the same pain pathways. It is therefore helpful to describe some general clinical features which point towards a non-mechanical diagnosis, and to describe some general laboratory tests which may be of value early, once suspicions have been raised. Of course, special tests are required to identify specific diseases, and these will also be discussed.

General features and laboratory investigation of suspected serious pathology

History

Non-mechanical causes of low back pain frequently have an insidious onset, although a minor traumatic event may be volunteered. Features characteristic of tumour, infection or central cord compression include continuous gnawing pain, night pain which prevents the onset of sleep and may lead to chair-resting, and a drawn facial appearance. Pallor, anorexia, weight loss, lassitude, fever, rigors and night-sweats should alert the clinician to a systemic pathology. Any back pain in a child should be taken seriously.

Examination

Abdominal, pelvic and flank examination may identify visceral pathology. Any swelling in the low lumbar or buttock region should raise suspicion of tumour or infection.

Investigations

In the presence of any of the above features, back pain should be urgently investigated. In general, a full blood count, serum electrolytes, bone biochemical screen (LFTs), erythrocyte sedimentation rate (ESR) and C-reactive protein will suffice to elicit systemic upset requiring specialist assessment.

Laboratory investigation of specific diagnoses in suspected serious pathology

Below are described features of non-mechanical back pain and associated laboratory tests which might reasonably be obtained by a general practitioner prior to (or at the same time as) referral of the patient to a specialist.

Spondyloarthropathy

Classically in young men, often associated with morning stiffness and episodic back pain, other large joints may be involved, especially the sacro-iliac joints.[1,2] Systemic symptoms may be evident, and there may be a history of uveitis or iritis, urethritis, psoriasis, inflammatory bowel disease or other gastro-intestinal upset.

Reiter's syndrome encompasses arthritis and uveitis in association with intestinal or genito-urinary symptoms. Urethritis requires a first catch urine specimen with specific request for *Chlamydia trachomatis* and *Neisseria gonorrhoea* culture. Serological evidence of recent infection is confirmed for *Chlamydia* in 20 per cent, and for *Yersinia* in a further 25 per cent.[3] Rheumatoid factor is positive in only 5 per cent of Reiter's syndrome, in contrast to 80 per cent of those with 'typical' rheumatoid arthritis.[4]

Ankylosing spondylitis is associated with 10–30% of Reiter's syndrome,[1] The spine is stiff, with costochondral and sacro-iliac joint involvement. Many develop hip or knee joint arthritis, and one third have iritis or inflammatory bowel disease. Rheumatoid factor is positive in 15 per cent, ESR is raised in 80 per cent and HLAB27 antigen is present in 95 per cent of white patients with this condition.[4]

Gout is rarely a cause of back pain.[1,5] Only 30 per cent of patients with gout will have elevated serum uric acid during an acute attack.[4] A moderate leucocytosis and elevated ESR occurs. Although joint aspiration and polaroid light examination for negatively birefringent crystals is more diagnostic, this is usually outside the remit of the general practitioner.

Infection

There are three main categories:

Vertebral osteomyelitis: primary (pyogenic or tuberculous) or secondary to a spinal procedure or other infective source such as pyelonephritis,[1] dental, respiratory or skin infections.[4]

Discitis: primary (junior school children are the commonest age) or secondary to intervertebral disc surgery or injection.

Epidural abscess: often associated with progressive neurology – a true spinal emergency.

Symptoms include pyrexia and weight loss. Muscle spasm is more marked and constant than in acute disc prolapse. Diabetics are at higher risk. Spinal infection is often diagnosed late, and may present with flank or abdominal pain.[6] Radiographs may be helpful, and ESR and white cell count are elevated. A tissue sample or aspirate should usually be obtained in the hospital under direct image control.

Neoplastic

Metastatic deposits are most frequent, usually with bony destruction. Common primary sites are breast, prostate, lung, thyroid and kidney. Pain tends to be constant, is unrelated to posture, increases in intensity and precedes the first radiographic changes.[7] ESR is likely to be elevated, and pancytopaenia reflects the degree of marrow involvement. Non-specific biochemical changes may include elevated alkaline phosphatase. If serum calcium is very high, parathyroid hormone will be suppressed, and this may help to discriminate primary hyperparathyroidism from hypercalcaemia of malignancy. Some neoplasms exhibit tumour markers such as prostatic specific antigen (PSA) which is markedly elevated in metastatic prostatic carcinoma and it is argued that this test should be done in men over 55 years of age.

Primary tumours are unusual in the adult spine. They may be benign (such as chordoma, meningioma, neurofibroma, eosinophilic granuloma, osteoid osteoma), haematological malignancies (myeloma, lymphoma, leukaemia), or sarcomas (Paget's osteosarcoma, chondrosarcoma, angiosarcoma). In children with leukaemia, non-specific back pain is one of the commonest presenting complaints. With the exception of the haematological disorders, laboratory tests fail to identify the specific neoplasm. In leukaemia and lymphoma there will be dramatic abnormalities in the blood count. In multiple myeloma, plasma and urine electrophoresis reveal monoclonal protein in 99 per cent. Urine is also analysed for Bence-Jones proteins, hyperalbuminuria and elevated urate excretion. Anaemia is found in 60 per cent and ESR is raised in 90 per cent.

Metabolic

Hyperparathyroidism may present with bone pain, abdominal cramps or renal colic. Laboratory tests which aid diagnosis must include serum calcium, phosphate, alkaline phosphatase and parathyroid hormone levels.

Guillain-Barré syndrome (acute infective neuritis) produces back pain, leg pain and weakness, which are easy to misdiagnose.[8,9] Multiple sclerosis often presents in a similar fashion. In Guillain-Barré syndrome, a history of acute respiratory or gastrointestinal illness may be elicited. Raised viral titres in serum are found. When hospitalized, lumbar puncture reveals elevated protein in cerebrospinal fluid.

Acute intermittent porphyria is rare, but one of the 'great mimickers'. Back and abdominal pain occur, together with bizarre neurological features. Levels of serum and urinary porphyrins and their precursors are elevated.

Visceral

Gynaecological

This group accounts for the largest number of patients with back pain after exclusion of spinal pathology. In the majority there is no inflammatory component and simple laboratory tests will be normal. Salpingitis, however, can precipitate symptoms of back pain and sacroiliitis. Appropriate high vaginal and endocervical swabs should be cultured.

Renal

Although ureteric pain in its classic form cannot be mistaken, acute pyelonephritis commonly presents as back pain. Dip-stick and standard mid-stream urine culture for bacteriuria should be performed. Organisms other than *Escherichia coli* may suggest a diagnosis of chronic pyelonephritis. Pseudomonas or proteus species are suspicious of anatomical abnormality of the urinary tract. Prostatitis, like salpingitis, leads to back pain and sometimes sacroiliitis. Rectal examination and urinary microbiology are helpful.

Pancreatitis

Sometimes a difficult diagnosis to make, serum amylase is usually elevated in an acute attack. In severe attacks, elevation of white cell count, blood glucose, serum lactate dehydrogenase and aspartate transaminase all occur early. Within 48 hours, serum calcium falls, haematocrit rises and arterial oxygenation is depressed. A metabolic acidosis may develop. In chronic pancreatitis, the pancreas is so attenuated that serum amylase may be normal. Laboratory evidence of malabsorption may be found.

Duodenal ulceration

Back pain is similar in quality to that in pancreatitis. In acute attacks, serum amylase may be mildly elevated, as may ESR and white cell count. *Helicobacter pylori* is associated with 95 per cent of chronic duodenal ulceration. Serological tests for this organism have 88 per cent sensitivity and 72 per cent specificity.

Vascular

Slowly dissecting aortic aneurysms produce acute back pain, and iliac vessel aneurysms may produce root compression symptoms. Abdominal examination and great vessel auscultation are essential to prevent misdiagnosis. Laboratory investigations are within the sphere of the acute hospital services.

Summary

It is vital for the primary healthcare physician to identify symptoms and signs of non-mechanical back pain. When this is suspected, simple laboratory tests, sometimes supplemented by more specific investigations allows a useful differential diagnosis to be achieved with speed.

References

1. Porter, R.W. (1993). *Management of Back Pain*. 2nd edn. Churchill Livingstone,.
2. Calin, A. (1979). Back pain: mechanical or inflammatory? *American Family Physician*, **20**, 97–100.
3. Wiesel, S.W. *et al*. (1996). *The Lumbar Spine*. 2nd edn. W.B.Saunders.
4. Wallach, D. (1996). *Interpretation of Diagnostic Tests*, 6th edn. Little Brown & Co.
5. Das De, S. (1988). Intervertebral disc involvement in gout: brief report. *J. Bone Joint Surg. [Br]*, **70B**, 671.
6. Flood, B.M., Deacon, P. and Dickson, R.A. (1983). Spinal disease presenting as acute abdominal pain. *Br. Med. J.*, **287**, 616–617.
7. Galasko, C.S.B. (1991). Spinal instability secondary to metastatic cancer. *J. Bone Joint Surg. [Br]*, **73B**, 104–108.
8. Turek, S.L. (1976). *Orthopaedic Principles and Their Applications*. Pitman Medical.
9. Winer, J. (1992). Guillain-Barré syndrome revisited. *Br. Med. J.*, **304**, 64–65.

Management

Chapter 14

Drug Therapy in Acute and Chronic Low Back Pain In Primary Care

Andrew Cole

Drug therapy is one of the many modalities of treatment available for the management of back pain. There is a vast array of drugs available and their varied use would suggest that there is no uniquely successful form of pharmacological therapy. Drug therapy does not alter the underlying condition causing the back pain but can modulate the important physiological effects of inflammation, muscle relaxation and central pain perception. However, the rationale for the use of a particular drug is often speculative and poorly supported by scientific evidence.

The purpose of this chapter is to present an overview of drug therapy in the primary care setting of patients with back pain in the absence of specific anatomical abnormalities. There have been four recent excellent reviews of the subject in the literature[1-4] and much of the information presented here is a synopsis of these. Interpretation of the available literature is problematic due to difficulty with diagnosis and poorly defined outcomes and any analysis must therefore take this into account.

Paracetamol

This is a member of the group of drugs classified as para-aminophenol derivatives. It has analgesic and antipyretic effects equivalent to those of asprin but it's anti-inflammatory effects are weaker. It acts by secondary inhibition of prostaglandin biosynthesis with a resultant increase in the pain threshold and modulation of the hypothalamic axis. Peak plasma levels occur after 30–60 minutes from ingestion.

It is effective against mild to moderate pain but its efficacy as an analgesic for severe pain is questionable. Because it is readily available the amount used, levels of satisfaction and efficacy remain conjectural.[2]

Paracetamol has a less favourable outcome when compared to NSAIDS[5] in the treatment of chronic back pain. Side effects include erythematous or urticarial rashes and hepatotoxity is a problem in overdose.

NSAIDS (Non-steroidal anti-inflammatories)

The primary mechanism of action of these drugs is a decrease in cyclo-oxygenase activity and a decrease in prostaglandin synthesis. Locally, NSAIDs reduce inflammation by inhibition of neutrophil function and the activity of phospholipase C. Pain relief may also be in part to a more central antinociceptive component. Several NSAIDs have been tested in clinical trials for low back pain and these generally show superiority over placebo therapy. Keos et al.[6] reviewed 26 randomized trials of NSAIDs and reached several conclusions;

- NSAIDs have good efficacy in acute back pain;
- They have only moderate efficacy in chronic back pain;
- NSAIDs are less effective in treating leg pain.

The anti-inflammatory activity of different NSAIDs is highly variable but patient differentiation of one particular NSAID against paracetamol or another reference drug is poor.[6] Therefore it is unlikely that one particular NSAID is better than another in terms of pain relief and the choice is best made on speed of action, half-life, duration of activity and patient tolerance.

The drawbacks of NSAIDs are well known and usually develop within the initial weeks of therapy. The incidence of side effects in combination with another NSAID is additive and there is little evidence to support any added benefit to the patient.

The development of selective COX 2 inhibitors theoretically provide a safer anti-inflammatory agent and there is some evidence that these are associated with a lower incidence of GI side effects.[7] The combination of misoprostaol and aspirin has also been shown to decrease the incidence of GI erosions.

Lipetz et al.[1] have suggested that NSAIDs are a reasonable first line choice for acute back pain with the majority of its effects being felt in the first week. Phenylbutasone is not currently recommended based on an increased risk of immunosuppression.

Muscle relaxants

This group includes a variety of pharmacologically different drugs including benzodiazepines, antihistamines and other sedatives. Their use is based on the supposition that muscle spasm is responsible for the pain, however this is disputed by many. In his recent overview of the literature Deyo[3] suggested that several of these medications were more efficacious than placebo and that their use is more effective in acute rather than chronic pain. In a further review, Von Feldt[2] agreed that muscle relaxants were better than placebo although the effects were often short lived and often failed to reach statistical significance.

The effect of the addition of a muscle relaxant to an NSAID remains unproven although a study by Cherkin et al.[8] found this to be a common practice. Muscle relaxants have gained a wide acceptance and at recommended doses these agents are generally well tolerated. Muscle relaxants and diazepam in particular have potential for abuse and chronic use should be avoided and should be limited to 1–2 weeks of pain symptoms.

Antidepressants

The commonly prescribed antidepressants are the tricyclic antidepressants (TCAs) and the selective serotonin re-uptake inhibitors (SSRIs). The TCAs work through a pre-synaptic inhibition of both noradrenaline and serotonin re-uptake. The SSRIs work at the same site but are selective in their action. The available literature is largely with the use of the TCAs in chronic pain syndromes. These agents are now believed to have a primary analgesic effect probably related to effects on monoamines in pain pathways.[9] Other suggested mechanisms have included their antihistamine properties, increased endorphin secretion and an increased density of cortical calcium channels.

There have been a few trials evaluating the efficacy of TCAs specifically for low back pain[10] but the results have been conflicting with high drop-out rates, however they can elevate mood and may increase pain tolerance.[11] The onset of analgesia with these agents may be delayed for up to 3 months. The newer SSRIs have not yet been fully evaluated for use in chronic pain syndromes although recently Atkinson *et al.*[12] in a double blind randomized study found them to be better than placebo but not as effective as noradrenergic antidepressants.

Occurrence of serious adverse side effects is low as the doses are generally lower than those given for depression.

This group of drugs remain useful adjuncts even though their analgesic mechanism remains unclear. They are generally not necessary in the management of acute low back pain.

Opioid analgesia

These drugs produce their analgesic effect by binding to opioid receptors displacing endogenous opioid compounds. (Mu, Kappa and Delta receptors). Morphine is the most commonly used and this occupies the Mu receptors both centrally and peripherally. The opioids commonly used include morphine, pethidine and the partial agonist buprenorphine.

The adverse effects of opioids can be a problem and the aim of successful administration will involve a balance of the analgesic effects against the adverse effects such as somnolence, confusion and constipation.

These drugs are frequently used for severe pain particularly in the setting of neoplastic disease.

In a review of medication for back pain Lipetz *et al.*[1] feel that the role of opioids in acute back pain is limited and that they should be reserved for those patients who have failed to gain adequate relief from other medications or in neoplastic disease. The prescribing doctor needs to be aware of the possibility of dependence although Schofferman[13] found that long-term opioid analgesic therapy was a reasonable option for severe refractory pain. It was well tolerated in patients who were carefully selected and had failed all other forms of therapy. Its use in chronic back pain syndromes has also been advocated by others who feel that there is no significant risk of abuse.[14]

Corticosteroids (oral)

These are typically prescribed for their anti-inflammatory activity but most have some mineralocorticoid activity. They regulate gene expression and subsequent protein synthesis in their target tissues. Through their action on phospholipase A2 they inhibit prostaglandin and leukotriene synthesis and decrease the inflammatory response at an earlier stage than the NSAIDS. They also have a direct action on the responses of lymphocytes and macrophages. Well-recognized complications include suppression of the pituitary–adrenal axis, electrolyte disturbance, hyperglycaemia and demineralization of bone. Many of these effects can be reduced by alternate day use but even short-term use of high dose steroids can contribute to cataract formation, myopathy, central nervous system disturbance and avascular necrosis of the femoral head. There are few studies investigating the use of oral steroids[15,16] and whilst they provide a theoretically useful anti-inflammatory agent their use in acute and chronic lumbar back pain remains unproven.

Local anaesthetics

These may be used for trigger point injections. However, the importance of trigger points remains controversial with low levels of reproducibility. There has been a randomized trial of local anaesthetic injection into trigger points[17] which failed to show any difference from placebo of needle insertion alone. The potential risks of injection include infection, nerve injury and haemorrhage.

Colchicine

Derived from the plant *Colchicum autumnale*, this drug interferes with the normal functioning of mitotic spindles. It results in an inhibition of metabolic and phagocytic activity of macrophages as well as decreasing the release of histamine from mast cells acting as a powerful anti-inflammatory. Its use has been advocated both orally and intravenously with anecdotal reports suggesting a positive effect on back pain. However, clinical trials would suggest that there is little benefit over placebo therapy[18,19] and it is therefore not commonly used in the management of back pain. It is contraindicated in patients with GI, renal, hepatic and cardiac disease.

Drug therapy in acute back pain

Recent guidelines have been published on the drug management of acute back pain.[20] To provide symptomatic relief during the period when natural recovery can be expected, the guidelines recommend use of acetominophen (paracetamol) and NSAIDS. Muscle relaxants and short course opioids were not generally recommended although were considered 'options' in more refractory cases. Because of the availability of equally effective alternatives they recommended against the use of opioids for more than 2 weeks. Oral steroids, colchicine and anti-depressants are not recommended for acute back pain.

Drug management of chronic back pain

The efficacy of drug therapy is generally less certain in this group of patients. Other factors such as socio-economic, psychological and medicolegal all have implications on the patient response to therapy. There are no published guidelines on the drug management although in a review of the subject by Von Feldt *et al.*[2] they suggested that combination analgesic therapy including paracetamol, NSAIDS, muscle relaxants and low dose opioids may be necessary. However there are few studies with regards to combination therapy in chronic low back pain.

Sleep disturbance is often associated with chronic back pain and low dose TCAs are a useful adjunct.

Summary

The study of the efficacy of the drug treatment of patients with back pain is difficult. There are problems with diagnostic difficulty and ambiguity and the outcome measures are often poorly defined. There are important psychological, social and cultural influences on the response to treatment all of which are difficult to allow for in clinical trials. Furthermore, a critical limitation of many trials is that they are conducted in referral centres where the patients are likely to be atypical and the findings largely irrelevant to general practice.[21]

All of these factors need to be taken into account when interpreting the literature.

Overall there is little science or clear evidence to guide us in the rational use of medications in back pain.

References

1. Lipetz, J.S. and Malanga, G.A. (1998). Oral medications in the treatment of acute low back pain. *Occup. Med.*, **13**(1), 151–166.
2. Von Feldt, J.M. and Ehrlich, G.E. (1998). Pharmacologic therapies. *Phys. Med. Rehabil. Clin. N. Am.*, **9**(2):473–487.

3. Deyo, R.A. (1996). Drug therapy for back pain. Which drugs help which patients? *Spine*, **21**(24), 2840–9; discussion 2849–2850.

4. Porter, R.W. and Ralston, S.H. (1994). Pharmacological management of back pain syndromes. *Drugs*, **48**(2),189–198.

5. Hickey, R.F. (1982). Chronic low back pain: a comparison of diflunisal with paracetamol. *New Z. Med. J.*, **95**(707), 312.

6. Koes, B.W., Scholten, R.J., Mens, J.M. and Bouter, L.M. (1997). Efficacy of non-steroidal anti-inflammatory drugs for low back pain: a systematic review of randomised clinical trials. *Ann. Rheum. Dis.*, **56**(4), 214–223.

7. Hayller, J. and Bjarnason, I. (1995). NSAIDS, COX-2 inhibitors and the Gut (Commentary). *Lancet*, **346**, 521–522.

8. Cherkin, D.C., Wheeler, K.J., Barlow, W. and Deyo, R.A. (1998). Medication use for low back pain in primary care. *Spine*, **23**(5), 607–614.

9. Magni, G. (1991). The use of antidepressants in the treatment of chronic pain. A review of the current evidence. *Drugs*, **42**(5), 730–748.

10. Turner, J.A. and Denny, M.C. (1993). Do antidepressant medications relieve chronic low back pain? *J. Fam. Pract.*, **37**(6), 545–553.

11. Ward, N.G. (1986). Tricyclic antidepressants for chronic low-back pain. Mechanisms of action and predictors of response. *Spine*, **11**(7), 661–665.

12. Atkinson, J.H., Slater, M.A., Wahlgren, D.R. *et al.* (1999). Effects of noradrenergic and serotonergic antidepressants on chronic low back pain intensity. *Pain*, **83**(2), 137–145.

13. Schofferman, J. (1999). Long-term opioid analgesic therapy for severe refractory lumbar spine pain. *Clin. J. Pain*, **15**(2), 136–140.

14. Jamison, R.N., Raymond, S.A., Slawsby, E.A., Nedeljkovic, S.S. and Katz, N.P. (1998). Opioid therapy for chronic noncancer back pain. A randomized prospective study. *Spine*, **23**, 2591–2600.

15. Green, L.N. (1975). Dexamethasone in the management of symptoms due to herniated lumbar disc. *J. Neurol. Neurosurg. Psychiat.*, **38**(12), 1211–1217.

16. Haimovic, I.C. and Beresford, H.R. (1986). Dexamethasone is not superior to placebo for treating lumbosacral radicular pain. *Neurology*, **36**(12), 1593–4.

17. Garvey, T.A., Marks, M.R. and Wiesel, S.W. (1989). A prospective, randomized, double-blind evaluation of trigger-point injection therapy for low-back pain. *Spine*, **14**(9), 962–964.

18. Schnebel, B.E. and Simmons, J.W. (1988). The use of oral colchicine for low-back pain. A double-blind study. *Spine*, **13**(3), 354–357.

19. Simmons, J.W., Harris, W.P., Koulisis, C.W. and Kimmich, S.J. (1990). Intravenous colchicine for low back pain: a double-blind study. *Spine*, **15**(7), 716–717.

20. Bigos, S., Bauyer, O., Braen, G. *et al.* (1994). Acute low back problems in adults. Clinical practice guideline No. 14. AHCPR Public No. 95–0642 Rockville,MD: Agency for health care policy and Research, Public Health Service, US Department Of health and Human Services.

21. Phillips, W. (1994). Drug therapy for back pain. Which drugs help which patients? *Spine*, **21**(24), 2840–9; discussion 2849–2850.

Chapter 15

Spinal Surgery

James Wilson-MacDonald

Surgery for back pain is indicated in only a small minority of patients, but even in highly selective patients the results can be quite variable, and surgery is not without possible complications. Surgery is only indicated in those who have failed an appropriate non-operative treatment programme. Patients must understand that the aim of surgery is improvement rather than abolition of pain. Recovery time from surgery is typically two to three months, and may be longer. Improvement in symptoms may continue for up to a year after the surgery.

Patients with nerve root compression pain in association with back pain tend to have better results than those undergoing surgery for back pain alone. Improvement in symptoms can occur in 80–85% of patients following surgery to stabilize a spondylolisthesis and to decompress nerve roots. The reasons for these individuals doing rather better are not clear.

Certain factors militate against a good result, particularly in those litigating for their back pain. Indeed surgery for back pain in those litigating is seldom indicated. Single level disease responds more favourably to surgery than multiple level disease, and surgery for back pain is seldom indicated at more than two levels.

Adverse prognostic factors

Litigation
Previous surgery – 'failed back'
Multiple level disease
Manual worker
Young male
Smoker
Psychosocial factors

Patient selection is very important. If psychological assessment suggests a lot of anxiety and stress, surgical results are less good. Waddell has described inappropriate signs which may suggest that pain is not organic in origin.[1] If this is the case, the pain is unlikely to respond well to surgical management.

Physical symptoms and signs which, when combined, point to the presence of non-organic factors in the production of back pain (Waddell signs):

1. Tenderness that is either superficial or non-anatomic in distribution or both.
2. Simulation of back pain stimulation by axial loading (pressure on the vertex of the erect subjector rotation of the pelvis and shoulders in the same plane avoiding spinal movement).
3. Discrepancies in 'straight leg raising test' performance in the sitting and supine positions.
4. Regional disturbance such as stocking distribution of hyperaesthesia or generalized weakness of a region.

Waddell signs (adapted with permission from Waddell: *The Back Pain Revolution*, Churchill Livingstone, page 162).[2]

Indications for surgery

Spinal surgery is usually indicated for the treatment of nerve root pain in the leg (sciatica) or for back pain, or for a combination of the two. Surgery for nerve root pain tends to be more successful than back pain surgery.

The most common indications for surgery for nerve root pain are:

1. Disc prolapse.
2. Spinal stenosis.

Rarer causes include tumours, infections, ganglia etc.

The main indication for surgery for back pain is for mechanical pain where the pain source can be accurately identified. The patients fall into three groups.

1. Discogenic back pain secondary to disc degeneration.
2. Spondylolisthesis where there is some bony defect leading to slippage between two vertebrae. This is often associated with nerve root signs and symptoms, such as leg pain, numbness and weakness.
3. Failed back surgery. The majority of these patients have had discectomy or decompression, although a minority may continue to experience back pain after attempts at fusion, and this occasionally is an indication for further surgery.

Clinical presentations

Disc prolapse

- Usually presents in the third and fourth decades of life.
- Episode of acute back pain is followed by nerve root pain.
- The back pain often improves when the nerve root pain starts.

- Nerve root pain is often accompanied by neurological signs and sciatic stretch test usually positive.
- Ninety per cent resolve within 6 weeks, the remainder may require invasive treatment.

Spinal stenosis

- Usually presents in the fifth decade of life or later.
- Usually insidious onset.
- Pain usually worst standing and walking (do not confuse with vascular claudication).
- Pain usually relieved by bending forward or sitting.
- There may be no abnormal signs on examination, including normal SLR.
- Commonest findings – absent ankle jerks, loss of lumbar lordosis.

Mechanical back pain

- Can occur in any adult – very common.
- Usually activity related.
- Pain usually relieved by rest.
- Clinical signs usually isolated to the back (stiffness, tenderness, spasm).
- Look for a spondylolisthesis (may see or feel a step in the spinous processes at L4/L5).

Tumours or infection

- Pain often constant.
- Pain not activity related.
- Night pain common.
- Tumours commoner in elderly.
- Is there any relevant history for tumour or infection (e.g. history of tumour, TB contact etc.).

Investigations

MRI scan is a very sensitive investigation for individuals with back disorders. It is important to be aware that with increasing age degenerative disc disease is normal, and can be considered part of normal ageing. Many younger individuals also experience early disc degeneration, and there is some evidence that this may be genetic in origin. Frequently multiple discs are affected by degeneration. The majority of these individuals are asymptomatic. Similarly although spondylolysis and spondylolisthesis are very common in the community (6 per cent of the population), it is seldom a significant source of pain. Therefore the presence of abnormalities on MRI scan should not be assumed to be the source of the symptoms. This is particularly true of older individuals.

MRI scans are also very useful for assessing nerve root and spinal cord compression either within the spinal canal or in the foramina where the nerves exit from the spinal canal.

The absence of any abnormality on MRI scan however, makes a mechanical cause of pain very unlikely indeed, and therefore MRI can usefully be used as a screening assessment. Surgery for back pain would almost never be indicated in those with a normal MRI scan.

CT scans are still useful sometimes. They are particularly good for assessing bone architecture, for example in a spondylolisthesis, and may be useful if there is a previous metal implant in place (although some distortion of the image invariably occurs). Occasionally this will be combined with a myelogram.

Myelography is rarely indicated now that MRI scanning is available. However if there is a metal implant in place, or some contra-indication to MRI scanning such as a pacemaker, myelography may occasionally be indicated.

Plain X-rays have little place in the management of spinal disorders, except for assessment of deformity. Where MRI is not available it may be useful to exclude tumour and infection, although it is not as sensitive.

Bone scanning can be useful in excluding infection or tumour.

Discography may be used to assess the pain source. Using local anaesthetic the disc or discs suspected of being the pain source are injected with a small volume of radio-opaque dye. A positive response is reproduction of the usual back pain of the patients when the dye is injected into the disc, and this helps the surgeon in deciding which levels of the spine to operate on.

Indications for surgery

The main indications for surgery to the spine (in order of frequency) are:

1. Compression of nerve roots or spinal cord with symptoms, including cauda equina syndrome.
2. Back pain.
3. Deformity.

Neurological compression

Compression of neurological structures can cause pain or neurological dysfunction. The pain is typically in the legs usually below the knees, in the distribution of a nerve root or multiple nerve roots. Neurological signs may include numbness in the legs, weakness or poor coordination. Patients may say that their legs feel unsteady or rubbery.

Symptoms of neurological compression may be improved by various measures other than surgery.

Waiting

Ninety per cent of those with disc prolapse will have resolution of their symptoms within 6 weeks, and even a proportion of those with spinal stenosis will find that their symptoms improve spontaneously.[3] The only contraindication to waiting is if there are deteriorating neurological signs such as weakness or more importantly signs of a cauda equina syndrome (perineal numbness, loss of bladder and bowel function).

Epidural steroid injection

This is mainly useful for controlling the pain of neurological compression, and will cure symptoms of perhaps 30 per cent of those with acute disc prolapse and 10 per cent of those with spinal stenosis. The procedure can be done as a day case under local anaesthetic, and can be repeated if helpful. It is sometimes used as a stop-gap for patients awaiting surgery, particularly in those with root symptoms but no radiological signs of compression.

Calcitonin injections

About 25 per cent of those with spinal stenosis will respond to injected calcitonin. This probably works as a vasodilator for the nerve root. It is most effective in the elderly and those with central stenosis, and is usually given as 16 injections over a four-week period.

This treatment may be offered as an alternative to surgery, particularly in high-risk patients. It can also be used as a stop-gap for those waiting for surgery.

Chemonucleolysis

This is a technique where the disc is injected with the enzyme, chymopapain, which denatures the proteins inside the disc and shrinks the disc to a smaller size. This technique is best in younger individuals where the disc is contained (it has not ruptured through the annulus). The procedure can be carried out as a day case and provided the indications are appropriate success rates of around 75 per cent should be achieved.[4] It cannot be repeated because of the danger of anaphylaxis due to development of hypersensitivity.

Discectomy

This is used for patients with a proven disc prolapse. The part of the disc pressing on the nerve root together with any other loose pieces of disc within the disc space are removed in order to take the pressure off the nerve root. Indications include failure of pain to resolve within 6 weeks, weakness or progression of symptoms. Results tend to be best in the young and in those with sequestrated disc prolapses (where the disc is free within the spinal canal). Success rates of around 90 per cent are widely reported.[5]

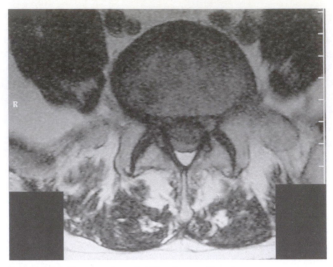

Figure 15.1 A left-sided disc hernia at L4/5 prior to discectomy.

Clinically, discectomy is best for pain relief, with improvement in muscle power being usually reasonable, but return of sensation is variable. In a study by Schade *et al.* (1999), it was reported that whilst significant disc herniation seen on MRI was an important predictor for a successful surgical outcome, rates of recovery and return to work were dependent on psychological factors, in particular work satisfaction.[6]

Surgery is usually carried out through a small incision posteriorly either by removing the ligamentum flavum alone, with a laminotomy (removal of part of the lamina) or with a laminectomy where the whole lamina is removed. Short-term results are best with the less invasive methods, but long term there is little difference.

The patients usually stay in hospital 3–5 days although it can be carried out as a day case procedure.

Spinal decompression

This operation is used to take the pressure off the nerve; discectomy is a type of decompression, but in spinal stenosis bone and soft tissues (mainly the ligamentum flavum) are removed through a posterior incision to release the nerves at the base of the spine. Surgery is successful in improving leg symptoms in about 70 per cent of those with spinal stenosis, and about 50 per cent will have some relief of back pain.[7] Patients are usually in hospital 4–7 days. Surgery is carried out through a posterior incision, and the extent of the procedure will depend on the number of levels requiring surgery.

Spinal stabilization

There are a number of different techniques available to stabilize the spine. The most commonly used is spinal fusion which is a joint arthrodesis.

Table 15.1 Average results of different techniques of surgical spinal fusion

Method	% Fusion rates	% Satisfactory outcome	% Unsatisfactory outcome
Anterior interbody (1072)	78	76	21
Posterior fusion (1264)	87	70	15
PLIF (1372)	89	82	11
PLF+Int Fix (463)	87	65	16
PLF+Ped screw (1125)	91	67	12
PLIF+Ped screw (305)	94	88	12

Other techniques have been developed such as devices which act like ligaments, or disc replacement which is similar to other joint replacements. Very variable results have been reported, but overall a success rate of about 70 per cent can probably be achieved,[8] success being improvement rather than abolition of pain. Those with nerve root compression or spondylolisthesis tend to have better results than other patients. It is in this group of patients that selection of the patient is most important, and those with inappropriate signs or adverse prognostic factors (see above) are probably best treated non-operatively. The MRC is currently sponsoring a randomized trial comparing surgery with rehabilitation.[9]

Table 15.1 summarizes the average results reported in the literature for the different techniques of spinal fusion.

Complications of surgery

Operations to fuse the spine are fairly major operations, and typically require a hospital stay of between five and 14 days. Patients should not undergo the surgery without appropriate preoperative counselling about the surgery itself, but also about the possible complications.

Pain

A proportion of patients experience increasing back pain following the surgery, for reasons which are not always clear. Some patients seem to develop pain not dissimilar to sympathetic dystrophy, and these patients are particularly difficult to treat. However, fortunately they are in a minority. I usually warn the patient that it will take two months to get over the operation and another month to two months to feel any really useful benefit from the surgery. In general improvement continues for up to a year after the operation.

Bone donor pain

Up to 50 per cent of patients develop significant pain from the bone donor site (usually the pelvis). Unfortunately man-made materials and allograft bone do not appear to result in such a high fusion rate as when the patient's own bone is used. However, the patient's bone can be mixed with allograft or man-made materials such as hydroxyapatite, and the fusion rates appear to be satisfactory using these techniques. The pain usually subsides in the months following surgery, although up to 25 per cent of patients may experience long-term pain from the bone donor site. However, if this is the case, it is seldom as severe as the preoperative back pain.

Infection

Fortunately deep infection at the site of surgery is unusual, but deep infection rates of up to 5 per cent are reported in certain papers, particularly where large posterior instrumentation is used. Infection can be a serious complication with the large implants (which are usually metal) used nowadays, and abscesses may require drainage. In general antibiotic treatment is recommended during the time that any implant is in place, and the implants may well require removal. However, in general the implants are usually left in place until such time as fusion has occurred, and they can then safely be removed. However, if the implants become seriously loose and are not effective, removal may be appropriate at an earlier stage. Removal of some infected metalwork, such as anterior cages, can be very difficult and present a serious risk to the patient.

Signs of post-operative infection include pain, fever, headache, photophobia (if meningism), swelling over the wound and drainage or leakage of fluid or pus (if fluid think of CSF).

Complications of surgery

Pain
Bone donor pain
Infection
Neurological damage
Non-union
Cutaneous nerve damage
Metalwork failure

Neurological damage

Approximately 2 per cent of individuals undergoing instrumentation using pedicle screws will develop long-term neurological symptoms. These may include leg pain, leg numbness or weakness, or very rarely damage to the cauda equina with bowel and urinary symptoms. In some cases the damage is reversible, and for example, removal of the pedicle screw pressing on a nerve root may result in satisfactory resolution of symptoms, but unfortunately in some individuals the symptoms are long term. Patients should always be warned about the risk of neurological damage prior to this type of surgery.

Non-union

Non-union is relatively common for example in non-instrumented spinal fusion, hence the development of instrumentation to increase fusion rates. Although non-union may be associated with a satisfactory clinical result, there is good evidence that those with unsatisfactory results have a higher non-union rate. This is one of the reasons why 360° fusion has increased in popularity, because it has a higher fusion rate. The success rates are also better. If the patient has a non-union, and continuing symptoms, there may be a case for considering revision surgery to improve the symptoms.

Cutaneous nerve damage

Cutaneous nerve damage is not uncommon particularly from the bone donor site. Posteriorly cluneal nerves passing over the posterior iliac wing can be damaged by posterior bone grafting techniques, particularly if a transverse incision is used. The lateral cutaneous nerve of the thigh can be damaged by anterior bone grafting techniques. These can result in painful neuromata, and can lead to persistent pain at the bone graft donor site.

Metalwork failure

Metalwork failure can occur, for example breakage of screws or rods, or dislocation of disc implants. In the majority of cases, this is either due to a failure of technique, or due to delayed union or non-union of the bone graft. These complications may require revision surgery. However even if there is broken metalwork or non-union, a good result can still be achieved.

The future

At the moment surgeons are concentrating on improving techniques which result in less morbidity and higher fusion rates. There is no doubt that the development of minimally invasive endoscopic surgery has reduced the morbidity for patients undergoing this type of surgery. It may be in the future that disc replacement surgery may result in better outcomes for selected patients with back pain.

Selection of appropriate patients for spinal fusion remains the main problem. It is not uncommon to see a patient with a perfectly fused spine with continuing or worsened symptoms following surgery. If surgeons can in some way improve selection techniques, much more reliable results might be obtainable.

Genetic engineering may provide exciting possibilities in the future. Bone-inducing proteins are already in experimental use to induce fusion, using much less invasive techniques than are used nowadays. Bio-technology may also provide the opportunity in the future for replacing the disc with a viable human disc, or by injecting material into a degenerate disc which somehow rejuvenates it.

The underlying causes of back pain are still poorly understood, and it may be possible in the future to find more accurate ways of pinpointing the pain source in patients.

Summary

Important points to remember are:

- patient selection is very important;
- patients should understand that the aim of the surgery is to improve pain rather than abolish it completely;
- surgery is less good in patients who smoke or those with psychosocial problems;
- abnormalities on scanning should not be presumed to be the cause of pain when considering surgery (surgery in the presence of a normal MRI is almost never indicated).

Surgery for back pain remains a challenge. Excellent results are achievable, but not reliably so. There are very few prospective random-ized trials assessing spinal fusion, and no trials which compare spinal fusion with physical treatments such as physiotherapy or rehabilitation. The Medical Research Council of Great Britain is currently undertaking such a trial, and this may provide some answers in the future.

References

1. Waddell, G., McCullouch, J.A. and Kummel E. (1980). Non-organic physical signs in low back pain. *Spine*, **5**, 117–125.
2. Waddell, G. (1998). *The Back Pain Revolution*. Churchill Livingstone.
3. Hakelius, A. (1970) Prognosis in sciatica: a clinical follow-up of surgical and non-surgical treatment. *Acta Orth. Scand.* (Suppl.), **129**, 1–76.
4. Javid, M.J., Norby, E.J., Ford, L.T. *et al.* (1983) Safety and efficacy of chymopapain in herniated nucleus pulposus with sciatica. Results of a randomized double-blind study. *JAMA*, **249**, 2489–2494.
5. Boos, M. and Davis, R.A. (1994) A long term analysis of 984 surgically treated herniated lumbar discs. *J. Neurosurg.*, **80**, 415–421.
6. Schade, V., Semmer, N., Main, C.J., Hora, J. and Boos, N. (1999). The impact of clinical, morphological, psychosocial and work-related factors on the outcome of lumbar discectomy. *Pain*, **80**(1–2), 239–249.
7. Silvers, H.R., Lewis, P.J. and Asch, H.L. (1993) Decompressive lumbar laminectomy for spinal stenosis. *J. Neurosurg.*, **78**, 695–705.
8. Turner, J., Ersek, M. and Herron, L. (1992). Patient outcomes after lumbar spinal fusions. *JAMA*, **268**, 907–911.
9. Fairbank, J., Frost, H. and Wilson-MacDonald, J. (1994). Proposals for a spinal stabilisation trial. *J. Bone Joint Surg. [Br].*, **76B**(Suppl. II & III), 135.

Chapter 16

Physical Therapy

Anthony Larcombe

Physical therapy is the mainstay of treatment for simple back pain and it is delivered by chiropractors, osteopaths and chartered physiotherapists.

The professions

Chartered physiotherapy is the most well known of the physical therapies in the UK because it is accessible through the NHS. Most chartered physiotherapists work in hospital outpatient departments or GP surgeries, but there are also significant numbers who work in the private sector. Physiotherapy training is based on a three year degree course with a broad curriculum encompassing specialities such as orthopaedics, geriatrics, general medicine and paediatrics. A number of physiotherapists have postgraduate qualifications in manipulation, a speciality which is not included in their undergraduate training.

Chiropractic and osteopathy were founded in the USA towards the end of the 19th century when medicine was relatively unadvanced. Both were based around the concept of manipulation, but the philosophy of the professions was very different. Chiropractic was founded by Daniel Palmer who believed that manipulation affected the nervous system, while Andrew Still, who founded osteopathy, believed that manipulation affected blood flow. Over the past 100 years the techniques and philosophies have slowly evolved and there is now less difference between the two professions.

In the UK, chiropractors and osteopaths work primarily in private practice and are only NHS-funded in localities where primary care groups or health authorities have purchased chiropractic or osteopathic services. Both professions have led the field of complementary medicine by forming statutory regulatory bodies, the General Chiropractic Council and General Osteopathic Council. These bodies maintain standards and regulate training in their respective professions.

The training for chiropractic and osteopathy is based on a four or a five year full-time degree course. The development of manipulative skills forms a central part of these courses, as this is the most common form of treatment performed by chiropractors and osteopaths. Unlike physiotherapy, which involves a broader spectrum of training, chiropractic and osteopathic degree courses specialize more in the diagnosis and treatment of the musculoskeletal system with less emphasis on other specialities. The early establishment of an osteopathy college, in 1917, has led to a greater number osteopaths (2500) than chiropractors (1200) in the UK, although an equal number of chiropractic and osteopathic colleges now exist.

Professional letters

Chartered physiotherapists   MCSP SRP
Chiropractors   DC, BSc Chiro, BapSc Chiro, DipChiro (varies according to training school)
Osteopaths   DO or BScOst

Treatments

Physical therapists use common treatment techniques, regardless of their professional background. Some observers argue that too much emphasis is placed on treatments such as manipulation or massage when a considerable proportion of the work carried out by these professionals is based around assessment, diagnosis and problem solving.

Each of the physical therapy professions place great emphasis on patient assessment and examination. Problems are identified and addressed so that all aspects of the patient are taken into account; lifestyle, work, family background, interests and health beliefs. Treatment is often aimed at addressing disability rather than impairment, with goals set for the patient. Continual re-assessment throughout the course of treatment ensures that these goals are met. Patients are thus encouraged to play an active part in their own rehabilitation.

All three professions use manual therapy techniques. Manipulation techniques involve both high velocity thrusts, used to free stiff joints, or gentler mobilization techniques which allow the therapist to graduate the level of force. Chartered physiotherapists favour the latter.

Each profession also uses exercise and soft tissue techniques, such as massage and trigger point therapy (massage or acupuncture applied to painful muscular points). Electrical therapy is still used by all professions, although some observers are concerned about the lack of supporting evidence for their use and the fact that they may give false hope to patients with high expectations of a 'techno-fix'.

After moderate analgesia and non-steroidal anti-inflammatory drugs (NSAIDs), the three main treatment approaches for simple back pain are manipulation, advice and exercises.

Manipulation

There are a large variety of different manipulative techniques. As the manipulative professions – chiropractic, osteopathy and manipulating physiotherapists – have developed, the techniques have become common to all three professions. There have been a number of randomized controlled trials to assess the effectiveness of manipulation, but many suffer from poor methodology.[1] Much of the good quality evidence relates to the effectiveness of manipulation for acute low back pain.[1,2]

The evidence review of the Royal College of General Practitioners (RCGP) guidelines[3] in 1999, stated that:

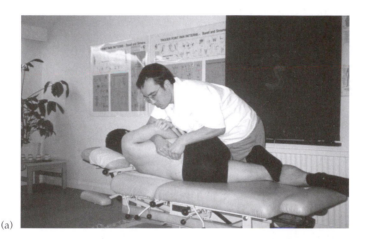

(a)

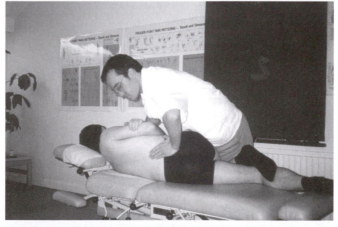

(b)

Figure 16.1 Examples of manipulation of the lumbar spine. (a) Short lever technique – applying force to each vertebra. (b) Long lever technique – applying force to pelvis to mobilize the lumbar spine.

'Within the first 6 weeks of onset of acute or recurrent low back pain, manipulation provides better short-term improvement in pain and activity levels and higher patient satisfaction than the treatments to which it has been compared.'

There is conflicting evidence from randomized controlled trials and systematic reviews for the efficacy of manipulation for chronic low back pain[2] and manipulation for radiculopathy is contraindicated, particularly in the presence of neurological signs. However lack of evidence does not imply that a technique does not work, only that it has not been shown to rigorously pass the test of randomized control trials. Many physical therapists feel that the judicious use of manipulation still has a role in the management of chronic back pain even though strong evidence to supports its use is lacking.

Risks and contraindications

The RCGP guidelines on acute low back pain advised that the risks of manipulation are very low when carried out by a trained practitioner.[4] Patients over 55 should be screened for osteoporosis, and malignancy if the patient's history raises any doubts of the integrity of the spine.

Advice and Information

The US Agency for Health Care Policy and Research (AHCPR),[5] UK Clinical Standards Advisory Group (CSAG)[6] and RCGP guidelines have carried out extensive, systematic reviews of the evidence and they have all strongly emphasized the importance of keeping active and avoiding prolonged bed rest following onset of acute low back pain. They also emphasize the importance of rehabilitation or reactivation of patients following an acute episode of back pain. This does not always mean teaching the patient exercises. Encouraging the patient to walk, swim and keep active are equally important.

Physiotherapists introduced Back Schools into the NHS several years ago. However these may have a greater role in the occupational setting.[7] Di Fabio (1995) concluded that Back Schools were most effective when coupled with a comprehensive rehabilitation programme.[8]

The physical therapist can encourage patients to remain active and thus reinforce any positive messages given to the patient by his or her GP. Treatment of the patient by most practitioners is not limited to the physical techniques. Educating the patient as to the cause of the problem, and giving relevant lifestyle advice, is also an essential part of the treatment. This should include specific ergonomic advice, particularly relating to posture, and the need to keep fit.

Exercises

The AHCPR, CSAG and RCGP guidelines state that mobility and exercise are indicated for patients with low back pain. Many practitioners take this a stage further by giving patients specific exercise programmes.

The large variety of exercises and the way that they are prescribed means that the research into their use has been very difficult to standardize. Some of this research suffers from poor methodology and many authors have called for better-designed trials to give a more accurate indication of which exercises are most beneficial. Faas (1996) concluded that specific exercises have no benefit in the management of acute low back pain but may be beneficial in treating patients with subacute or chronic low back pain.[9] There is no consensus on whether flexion exercises, e.g. William's exercises, are better than extension exercises, the latter often used as part of the McKenzie regime.[10–12]

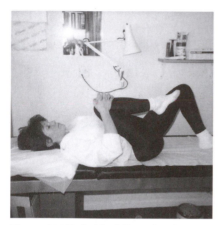 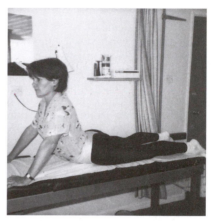

Figure 16.2 Individual flexion and extension exercises for the lumbar spine.

There is evidence to support the use of specific exercises in patients with subacute low back pain (6–12 weeks) and chronic low back pain (more than 12 weeks). Frost *et al.* (1995) found that supervised aerobic exercise programmes helped reduce disability and improve function in patients with chronic low back pain.[13] This study was further supported by Klaber-Moffet *et al.* (1999) who demonstrated that community-based exercises can help people suffering from subacute low back pain.[14]

Recent research[15,16] has identified weakness in the deep trunk musculature as a potentially important factor in the genesis of recurrent non-specific low back pain. Exercises have been developed by a number of physical therapists in this respect and the Pilate's technique is widely considered to help rehabilitate these important muscle groups.

Other physical therapy treatments

van Tulder et al. (1997) undertook a systematic review of interventions for acute and chronic low back pain.[7] They found that TENS, EMG biofeedback and acupuncture were no more effective than placebo, waiting list or other conservative treatments. Back Schools may be effective in an occupational setting.

There is little evidence to support the use of traction for simple low back pain.[17,18]

When to refer to a physical therapist

The trend for evidence-based medicine and the consensus of three comprehensive clinical guidelines has led to a widely agreed approach to the management of non-specific low back pain among the different professions. This approach is summarized in Table 16.1.

Once low back pain has been triaged by the GP as simple back pain, moderate analgesia and NSAIDs should be used for the first 1–3 weeks, in conjunction with advice to stay as active as possible and avoid bed rest. If there is no improvement within two weeks then referral to a chiropractor, osteopath or chartered physiotherapist is indicated. The early referral of patients whose pain does not improve is important to prevent the development of chronic pain and disability.

Patients need to be reassessed 6 weeks after the onset of symptoms, either by the GP or therapist. There should be particular vigilance for pathological red flags or psychosocial yellow flags (beliefs or behaviours on the part of the patient which may predict poor outcomes) in those patients who have not improved. Rehabilitation or aerobic reconditioning may be useful to implement if these flags are absent. Patients appearing to be developing long-term disability need to be referred to a specialist physician.

The guidelines have proposed this model of clinical management. The complete reviews of the evidence for these guidelines, and the assessment of the quality of that evidence, underlines that this is the modern approach to the treatment of simple back pain.

Table 16.1 A timetable for managing acute low back pain

DURING FIRST WEEK AFTER THE ONSET OF THE PAIN
General practitioner or practice physical therapist to perform diagnostic triage. For simple low back pain prescribe moderate analgesia and NSAIDs and give advice and reassurance. *The Back Book* (ISBN 011 702 0788) provides simple, straightforward advice for patients.

IF NO IMPROVEMENT AFTER TWO WEEKS
Refer to chiropractor, osteopath or physiotherapist for assessments and treatment e.g. manipulation (UK: Patients should be encouraged to use non-NHS practitioners if local resources do not allow rapid access to NHS physiotherapy. NHS providers should consider purchasing services from local non-NHS providers).

IF NO IMPROVEMENT AFTER 6 WEEKS OF PHYSICAL TREATMENT
Reassessment of the patient. Assess for red or yellow flags. Refer to appropriate specialist if either flags are present. Otherwise the patient should undergo rehabilitation or aerobic reconditioning.

Conclusion

Physical therapists have an important role in the management of patients with low back pain, particularly in avoiding chronic disability. Physiotherapists are well established in the British National Health Service and most state health systems around the world. Osteopaths and chiropractors are also now part of the mainstream health system and these professions are leading the field in the management of patients with mechanical low back pain.

References

1. Koes, B.W., Assendelft, W.J., van der Heijden, G.J. and Bouter, L.M. (1996). Spinal manipulation for low back pain. An updated systematic review of randomised clinical trials. *Spine*, **21**(24), 2860–2871; discussion 2872–2873.
2. Shekelle, P. (1995). Spinal manipulation and mobilisation for low back pain. Paper presented to the International Forum for Primary Care Research on Low Back Pain. Seattle October 1995.
3. RCGP. (1996). *Clinical Guidelines for the Management of Acute Low Back Pain*. September 1996. Royal College of General Practitioners, London.
4. Haldeman, S. and Rubinstein, S.M. (1992). Cauda equina syndrome in patients undergoing manipulation of the lumbar spine. *Spine*, **17**, 1469–1473.
5. AHCPR. (1994). *Clinical Practice Guidelines No. 14. Acute Low Back Problem in Adults*. December 1994. AHCPR Publication No. 95–0642. Agency for Health Care Policy and Research, Public Health Service, US Department of Health and Human Services, Rockville, MD.
6. CSAG. (1994). *Clinical Standards Advisory Group Report on Low Back Pain*. December 1994. HMSO.
7. van Tulder, M.W., Koes, B.W. and Bouter, L.M. (1997). Conservative treatment of acute and chronic nonspecific low back pain: a systematic review of randomized controlled trials of the most common interventions. *Spine*, **22**(18), 2128–2156.
8. Di Fabio, R.P. (1995). Efficacy of comprehensive rehabilitation programs and back school for patients with low back pain: a meta-analysis. *Phys. Ther.*, **75**(10), 865–878.
9. Faas, A. (1996). Exercises: which ones are worth trying, for which patients, and when?. *Spine*, **21**(24), 2874–2878.
10. Elnaggar, I.M., Nordin, M., Sheikhzadeh, A., Parnianpour, M. and Kahanovitz, N. (1991). Effects of spinal flexion and extension exercises on low-back pain and spinal mobility in chronic mechanical low-back pain patients. *Spine*, **16**(8), 967–972.
11. Delitto, A., Cibulka, M.T., Erhard, R.E., Bowling, R.W. and Tenhula, J.A. (1993). Evidence for use of an extension-mobilization category in acute low back syndrome: a prescriptive validation pilot study. *Phys Ther.*, **73**(4):216–22; discussion 223–228.
12. Stankovic, R. and Johnell, O. (1990). Conservative treatment of acute low-back pain. A prospective randomized trial: McKenzie method of treatment versus patient education in 'mini back school'. *Spine*, **15**(2), 120–123.
13. Frost, H., Klaber Moffett, J.A., Moser, J.S. and Fairbank, J.C. (1995). Randomised controlled trial for evaluation of fitness programme for patients with chronic low back pain. *BMJ.*, **310**(6973), 151–154.
14. Klaber-Moffett, J.A., Torgerson, D., Bell-Syer, S. *et al.* (1999). Randomised control trial of exercise for low back pain: clinical outcome, costs and preferences. *BMJ*, **319**, 279–283.
15. Hides, J.A., Stokes, M.J., Saide, M., Jull, G.A. and Cooper, D.H. (1994). Evidence of multifidus wasting ipsilateral to symptoms in patients with acute low back pain. *Spine*, **19**, 165–172.

16. Hides, J.A., Richardson, C.A. and Jull, G.A. (1996). Multifidus muscle recovery is not automatic following resolution of acute first episode low back pain. *Spine*, **21**(23), 2763–2769.
17. Beurskens, A.J., de Vet, H.C., Koke, A.J. *et al.* (1995). Efficacy of traction for non-specific low back pain: a randomised clinical trial. *Lancet*, **346**(8990), 1596–1600.
18. van der Heijden, G.J., Beurskens, A.J., Koes, B.W., Assendelft, W.J., de Vet, H.C. and Bouter, L.M. (1995). The efficacy of traction for back and neck pain: a systematic, blinded review of randomized clinical trial methods. *Phys. Ther.*, **75**(2), 93–104.

Chapter 17

The Role of the Specialist Physiotherapist

Patrick Hourigan

Striking changes in orthopaedic surgery have taken place in the past 30 years. The advances in techniques of joint replacement and trauma management have resulted in a substantial increase in the workload for orthopaedic surgeons, but this extra burden has not always been accompanied by an increase in human resources. Referrals from GPs seeking a specialist opinion for patients with mechanical low back pain continue to rise relentlessly.

In the late 1980's Robin Ling, an orthopaedic surgeon working in Exeter, recognized this dilemma, and instituted a system of managing his orthopaedic caseload whereby a physiotherapist saw a large proportion of the patients referred for an orthopaedic opinion. He recognized that physiotherapists were well trained in musculoskeletal examination techniques, and that with additional training could successfully manage a large proportion of patients who did not require surgical intervention.

Byles and Ling[1] published a survey of this system of patient management in 1989. They described the physiotherapist working as a first line filter system for orthopaedic referrals in which only 33 per cent of patients were actually passed to the orthopaedic surgeon, with most of these being listed for surgery. The remainder were independently managed by the physiotherapist. Eighty-eight per cent of the patients were satisfied with the management received, as were 80 per cent of the general practitioners (GPs). The practice was discontinued after Ling's retirement.

In 1992 the waiting time for a routine orthopaedic spinal opinion in the Exeter area was 18 months, with the routine waiting list for spinal surgery exceeding 2 years. Such long waiting times proved unsatisfactory to both GPs and patients, and clinics were struggling to fit in additional emergency patients, which led to the question: does a surgeon need to see every case of spinal pain referred to the clinic? This issue is particularly relevant when one considers that the number of patients needing surgery is only a small percentage of the total number of cases seen.

A physiotherapist with extensive experience of musculoskeletal medicine was appointed to work alongside the spinal surgeon and to review patients on his behalf. The physiotherapist underwent a period of training in the principles of spinal surgery, diagnosis and the management of broader medical conditions.

The physiotherapist assessed and examined patients in the orthopaedic out-patient clinic and arranged plain X-rays as necessary. Each patient was provided with a management plan, these being discussed with the surgeons in a weekly meeting.

The management plan consisted of one of the following:

- request for specialist radiological investigation, e.g. MRI;
- patient listed for surgery;
- patient passed over to consultant for diagnostic clarification;
- patient referred for conservative treatment;
- injection therapy arranged (epidural or apophyseal joint infiltrations.);
- patient referred on to other clinical specialist.

Only 24 per cent of cases seen by the physiotherapist were subsequently seen by the orthopaedic surgeon, with half of these being fast-tracked into surgical management. The physiotherapist also identified non-mechanical conditions, including spinal cord tumour, ankylosing spondylitis, and peripheral joint arthritis and these were referred to an appropriate physician.

The benefits of this system were:

- a fast-track service for surgical candidates;
- shortening of the waiting time for out-patient appointments;
- correct referral of patients wrongly assigned to the spinal clinic.

Initial outcomes of the first 100 patients seen by the physiotherapist were favourable.[2]

Similar projects began across the United Kingdom. By 1998, 43 centres had adopted a similar approach to the management of spinal disorders. Results of a national survey[2] consistently showed that only 25 per cent of cases referred into orthopaedic departments ultimately needed to see a surgeon. Substantial reductions in out-patient waiting times were also reported as a major benefit of this practice.

A survey[3] of the consultants working with the physiotherapists in these extended roles has outlined their approval of the practice, with 96 per cent declaring themselves satisfied or highly satisfied with the physiotherapists in the clinic role. Eighty-five per cent of the consultants confirmed that patients were waiting a shorter time for out-patient appointments, with 16 per cent of consultants reporting that they were able to spend more time in the operating theatre as a result of the physiotherapist seeing patients on their behalf.

More recent evidence has further supported the use of physiotherapists reviewing patients on behalf of doctors. Daker-White et al.,[4] in a randomized controlled trial in Bristol, compared the results and outcomes of patients seen in orthopaedic clinics-with about half the patients seen by a sub-consultant, post-fellowship doctor, and half seen by an experienced physiotherapist. Analysis of the results showed no significant difference in the outcomes of both groups, except in two areas; patient satisfaction was much greater and direct hospital costs lower in patients seen and managed by the physiotherapists.

Harrison[5] has expressed concern that the options for management may be limited if patients are not seen by a doctor. Will patients be denied the potential benefits of injection therapy? Such concerns are unfounded. Physiotherapists who have undergone additional post-graduate training are now performing intra-articular and peri-articular injections. In its Review of Prescribing of Medicines Report,[6] the Department of Health also recommends that physiotherapists should be allowed to prescribe from a limited number of drugs, particularly those working in such extended roles. Appropriate training would be given and competency will be ensured.

The physiotherapists involved in these specialist roles have formed a national Clinical Interest Group, The Extended Scope Practitioners (this name reflecting the substantial alteration in clinical practice of those involved). The group provides a peer support network, advise on the setting up of similar posts and a commitment to establishing a training programme to ensure the competency of physiotherapists progressing into such roles.

The specialist physiotherapist in primary care

Since such a large proportion of patients presenting at orthopaedic clinics have been inappropriately referred, could they be managed in another way? Hattam and Smeatham[7] have outlined the use of a specialist physiotherapist in primary care to screen patients for orthopaedic referral before they are sent to tertiary care centres. Of patients who would have been sent to hospital, Smeatham and Hattam managed 72 per cent of cases in primary care, obviating the need for hospital referral. If such practice were expanded with similar results, it could have a striking impact on reducing costs and cutting hospital waiting lists.

The challenge ahead is to encourage more specialist physiotherapists in primary care. Their potential role in supporting GPs in managing patients with low back pain has yet to be established. Important differences exist between hospital-based physiotherapy clinicians and those working directly with GPs. Radiological and orthopaedic support for specialist physiotherapists outside the hospital setting is vital for both training and maintaining high standards of diagnosis and orthopaedic management.

Specialist physiotherapists are ideally suited to provide secondary triage support to GPs in the primary care setting. They are well versed in orthopaedic investigations, and with the right training can request imaging and perform injections. They can provide conservative care for low back pain patients and are able to identify those that require surgery. They have the potential to greatly improve the management of patients with low back pain in Great Britain.

References

1. Byles, S.E. and Ling, R.S.M. (1989). Orthopaedic out-patients – a fresh approach. *Physiotherapy.* **75**(7), 435–437.

2. Hourigan, P.G. and Weatherley, C.R. (1994). Initial assessment and follow-up by a physiotherapist of patients with back pain referred to a spinal clinic. *J. Roy. Soc. Med..* **87**. 213–214.
3. Hourigan, P.G. and Weatherley, C.R. (1999). *Physiotherapists in Orthopaedic Clinics – Consultant Survey.* Horizon (The Extended Scope Practitioners Newsletter.) No. 4. February 1999.
4. Daker-White, G., Carr, A.J., Harvey, I. *et al.* (1999). A randomised controlled trial. Shifting boundaries of doctors and physiotherapists in orthopaedic out-patient departments. *J. Epidemiol. Commun. Health*, **53**, 643–650.
5. Harrison, M. (1999). Acute back pain needs attention; Letter. *Hospital Doctor*, **28/10/99**, 18.
6. Department. of Health. (1999) *Review of Prescribing, Supply and Administration of Medicines – Final Report*. March 1999.
7. Hattam, P. and Smeatham, A. (2000). Evaluation of an orthopaedic screening service in primary care. *J. Clin. Governance*, (in press).

For information on the Back Pain Triage Clinic at the Nuffield Orthopaedic Centre, Oxford go to: http://www.osrg.com/index1.htm

Epilogue

Implementation of RCGP Guidelines

Christine A'Court

This chapter summarizes the development and content of the Royal College of General Practitioners (RCGP) guidelines for the management of acute low back pain, and the success or otherwise with which they have been implemented in the UK. It then applies what is known about changing professional practice to implementation of these guidelines and aims to give readers ideas for effective approaches in their own geographic region.

Background to production of RCGP guidelines

Back pain is the single largest cause of time off work, and the associated disability claims are escalating. The social and financial cost underlies recent drives to improve the overall management of acute back pain. In 1996, the NHS Executive commissioned from the RCGP guidelines for the management of acute low back pain, based on a systematic review of evidence used in the 1994 reports of the Agency for Health Care Policy and Research (AHCPR) (US) and the Clinical Standards Advisory Group (CSAG) (NHS), plus evidence published subsequently.[1] In October 1996, a copy of the guidelines, together with an evidence-based patient self-help booklet called *The Back Book* was sent to every GP in the UK.[2] The development process and format of the guidelines satisfied rigorous standards defined elsewhere.[3,4]

The broad emphasis of these guidelines is that the management of acute low back pain should change from secondary to primary care, from rest to activity, and from a medical to multidisciplinary model, which may involve back care specialists currently operating primarily outside the NHS. A further important concept – the need for recognition of psychosocial risk factors for chronicity ('yellow flags'), was emphasized in the April 1999 update of the guidelines.

The underlying presumption, for which evidence has begun to accrue,[5] is that early, active management as advocated in the RCGP guidelines can reduce the disability and cost associated with both acute and chronic back pain.

Summary of RCGP guidelines

- Initial diagnostic triage should distinguish between mechanical back pain, nerve root compression, and patients with 'red flag' symptoms/signs indicating underlying pathology requiring investigation and/or referral.
- During triage efforts should also be made to identify patients with 'yellow flag' psycho-social features placing them at high risk of chronicity.
- Lumbar X-rays are rarely of value and represent a significant radiation dose.
- Outcome is improved if patients are advised to maintain normal activities; to not take bed rest (unless unavoidable, in which case it should be for no longer than 48 hours); and if analgesics are required these should be simple analgesics prescribed on a regular rather than 'as required' basis to help maintain mobility and avoid demoralizing resurgence of pain.
- Treatments associated with more risk than benefit are: traction, plaster jackets, manipulation under anaesthesia, benzodiazepines for >2 weeks and systemic steroids. Treatments providing some symptom relief but no impact on outcome include: analgesics, muscle relaxants, heat/cold, short wave diathermy, trigger point and epidural injections and lumbosacral girdles. Specific back exercises during acute pain show no clear benefit over normal activities.
- Within 6 weeks of onset, manipulation by a suitably trained practitioner is of low risk, and associated with a better outcome than treatments to which it has been compared.
- If pain persists more than 6 weeks, diagnostic triage should be repeated, due account taken of psychosocial factors maintaining debility, and patients referred for reactivation/rehabilitation. Exercise programmes and physical reconditioning produce some benefit to pain and functional level in chronic LBP, and should be started by 6 weeks. The evidence is inconclusive that manipulation produces clinically significant improvement in chronic LBP.

Are the RCGP guidelines changing practice? If not, why not?

In Britain, many GPs do not recall receiving or reading the RCGP guidelines, illustrating the perennial problem of paper overload, and the need for local implementation of national guidelines. Statistics from the Department of Health suggest that between 1996 and 1998, there was little change in prevalence of back pain and associated disability.[6] Taking this measure together with the impression of professionals in the field, it would seem that, to date, the impact of the guidelines has been rather limited.

Prior to the RCGP guidelines there was a dearth of guidance for GPs on best management of patients with acute back pain, although these patients comprise up to 9 per cent of consultations. Most doctors will agree that back pain was given little emphasis in the undergraduate curriculum, and may recall no training in anything other than acute disc prolapse and some of the relatively infrequent causes of back pain. Three regional pre-implementation audits conducted between 1996 and 1998 showed that 'red flag' symptoms and signs were acted upon appropriately by almost all GPs.

However, up to 47 per cent of GPs would request a lumbar X-ray for acute LBP, up to 66 per cent of GPs recommended bed rest, and 36 per cent advised against normal activities. Although around 65 per cent of patients had simple analgesia prescribed, it was to be taken on an 'as required' basis in 50 per cent. Few patients were referred for physiotherapy or manipulative treatment early in the course of back pain.

The RCGP guidelines have been heralded as both useful and long overdue, although some points, notably the recommendation for early manipulation, provoked controversy. This latter point may be one reason why GP's practice has been slow to change, since if professionals find one highly publicized issue hard to accept, it tends to mar their acceptance of the overall package. A single problematic point undermines confidence in the whole guidelines and seemingly offers an excuse for the practitioner to carry on as before.

The slowness with which professionals change long-established practice is a more general problem which is increasingly recognized. As stated in a 1999 Effective Health Care bulletin:[7]

> *'The naïve assumption that when research information is made available it is somehow accessed by practitioners, appraised, then applied in practice is now largely discredited. Whilst knowledge of a research-based recommendation or practice-based guideline is important it is rarely, by itself, sufficient to change practice.'*

There is a growing body of research into the changing of professional practice which should be of interest to all health professionals, whether orthodox or 'complementary'. The current chapter applies what is known about changing practice to the RCGP guidelines. It helps to first recognize the general distinction between *dissemination* and *implementation* of guidelines.[7]

Dissemination of guidelines, as attempted in 1996 by the mailing of guideline leaflets to all 65 000 UK GPs, is necessary to raise awareness of research messages, but is rarely of itself sufficient to change practice. In recent years there has been an exponential rise in the number of guidelines, of varying quality, issued to all NHS professionals. GPs receive most, by virtue of the breadth of their medical practice. A study conducted in Cambridge and Huntingdon found that in 32 practices a total of 855 separate guidelines had been retained for future reference.[4] So, as Phil Hammond the medical satirist says,

> *'. . . there are thousands of the damn things, and doctors differ in their ability to recall which drawer they put them in. So either you can't find them at all, or you end up treating angina with the irritable bowel guidelines. . .'.[8]*

So dissemination alone, although useful for awareness-raising, is generally insufficient. There is a need for *implementation* – a term to cover getting the findings adopted into practice with the required change in the professional's behaviour. As to how implementation is best achieved, the broad conclusions from reviews of multiple studies conducted between 1995 and 1998 are as follows;

• there are no 'magic bullets';
• a range of interventions are effective under some circumstances, but none is effective under all circumstances;
• success is more likely if interventions are broad-based and multi-faceted (more than two approaches) – with cost implications;
• interventions which address specific barriers to change are more likely to be effective;
• adequate resources are essential for effective implementation.

Strategies for implementation of RCGP guidelines

'Changing clinical practice seldom entails a single action, but usually demands a combination of different interventions, and recognition (preferably in advance) of obstacles to change.' (Grol, 1997)

Centralized lectures

A common approach to continuing medical education, the lecture, is rather discredited as a method of implementing change, but nonetheless has some value. At the very least lectures raise awareness of, for instance, the fact that there is now evidence-based guidance on management of acute back pain.

The efficacy of lectures is increased if they deal with specific barriers to change. The approach to implementation taken in Oxfordshire involved multidisciplinary 3-hour meetings entitled 'Back Pain – Controversy and Consensus', to which local GPs, physiotherapists, chiropractors, osteo-paths, relevant consultants and local fitness instructors were invited. A high turn out indicated considerable interest in back pain, and in a cross-professional approach.

The training sessions focussed on potential barriers to implementation as identified during a prior period of national and local consultation (see Box 1). Speakers included a few secondary care specialists (orthopaedic, neurosurgical or rheumatological). Their public endorsement of the RCGP guidelines was probably important for GPs in particular (see below, use of opinion-leaders). A follow-up questionnaire (Box 2) suggested the general approach was reasonably successful, although it must be acknowledged that without a RCT, there is a risk of over-estimating the impact.[7]

Box 1: Issues to be addressed during educational sessions on RCGP guidelines

• training/revision in effective diagnostic triage
• belief that back pain benefits from rest and that hurt always means harm

- dangers of medicalizing back pain with inappropriate investigations or 'labelling'
- value, limitations and disadvantages of various analgesic regimes
- appropriate and inappropriate referrals to secondary care services
- training and funding of local NHS physiotherapists
- sources of good patient information
- consumerism and usage of chiropractic and osteopathy
- GMC view on referrals by medical practitioners to non-medical practitioners
- voluntary and statutory registration of osteopaths and chiropractors
- view of medical defence organisations about cross-professional referrals
- role of the fitness industry in prevention and treatment of back pain
- strength of evidence base for various recommendations

Box 2: Follow-up questionnaire after educational evenings, 'Back Pain-Controversy and Consensus' held by Oxfordshire MAAG. Questionnaire was sent out to 106 attendees. Response rate 71 per cent

Q1.   How confident do you feel about distinguishing mechanical low back pain from nerve root pain or pain of a sinister nature ?
A1.   More confident (70%); the same (30%); less confident (0%)
Q2.   In acute apparently mechanical back pain (<6 weeks duration), how likely are you to avoid requesting an X-ray?
A2.   More likely (32%); the same (56% – most commented already aware of limited value); less likely (8%)
Q3.   How likely are you to recommend that a patient with acute mechanical back pain stays active and avoids bed rest, and if unavoidable, rests for no more than 48 hours?
A3.   More likely (56%); the same (41%); less likely (3%)
Q4.   In a patient with mechanical back pain persisting up to 6 weeks, how likely are you to refer to, or recommend the services of a registered manipulative therapist e.g. physiotherapist with suitable postgraduate training, chiropractor or osteopath? (responses from GPs shown)
A4.   More likely (50%); the same (45%); less likely (5%)
Q5.   In a patient with one or more episodes of mechanical back pain how likely are you to recommend general conditioning exercise to start when in remission, for possible prevention or minimisation of future episodes?
A5.   More likely (61%); the same (36%); less likely (0%)
Q6.   In a patient with back pain of less that 6 weeks duration how likely are you to manage without referral to secondary care (orthopaedics, neurosurgery or rheumatology)?
A6.   More likely (21%); the same (71%); less likely (3%)
Q7.   How likely are you to supply written information on acute back pain?
A7.   More likely (55%); the same (45%); less likely (0%)

Use of opinion-leaders

Research concerning the effectiveness of opinion-leaders to promote change finds mixed effects.[7] In Oxfordshire, the widespread support from relevant consultants for the RCGP guidelines is an important source of confidence for local GPs. By contrast, in Essex, for instance, at least one consultant specifically refused to endorse referral to chiropractors or osteopaths, which may well have inhibited GPs from increasing use of this resource. It may be of interest to hear the view of Neil Marshall, Standards Section of GMC, April 1998 that

> *'The days of doctors trying to ensure that only they treat patients are long gone.'*

This represents quite a turn around from the days when association with non-registered medical practitioners was viewed as gross professional misconduct!

Educational out-reach visit

An out-reach visit is where a trained person meets with practice professionals in their practice setting, with the intention of changing their performance.[7] Evaluation of this approach has been undertaken mainly in North America where it was found to be effective for changing prescribing practice. The limited uptake of local practice-based multi-disciplinary education on the back pain guidelines in Oxfordshire probably reflects the low priority given by many GP practices to the subject, and the perceived difficulties of tying up many clinical staff for training during the working day.

Reminder systems

Patient-specific reminder systems, either manual or computerized have been found to improve provision of preventive care, clinical management, and aid selection of drug dosages, but do not appear to improve diagnosis. In the absence of computerized decision support or protocols, GPs have to think of checking, and be able to find a copy, or remember the content of the RCGP guidelines when seeing a patient with acute back pain.

Audit and feedback

Another approach to changing professional practice is audit and feedback for which available evidence suggests a small-to-moderate effect only, at least when audit is imposed by parties extraneous to the practitioners.[7] Feedback alone has been used by Oxfordshire hospital's radiology departments who reply to a request for a lumbar X-ray for the assessment of acute back pain with a comment about the lack of appropriateness of the investigation for this clinical indication, and even a refusal to carry out the X-ray in the absence of clinical information justifying the request. Anecdotally, this appears to have a salutary effect on GPs' test-ordering!

If GPs within a practice decide they want to audit any aspect of their management, this will be made easier if they first ensure consistent recording of consultations, preferably using a limited number of appropriate Read codes (see Box 3).

Audits carried out by Camden and Islington MAAG (see Box 4) before and after educational meetings about the RCGP guidelines show gains in the right direction, some quite impressive, some rather small. These audit findings serve to emphasize how individual approaches to implementation tend to have a limited impact on practice. It is possible that the education offered did not address all the obstacles to change perceived by local health professionals.

Box 3: Consistent recording of back pain consultations using Read codes

Where GPs are Read-coding their consultations, then practices (and ideally, primary care groups) should identify a preferred code to facilitate future patient searches (e.g. to assess level of demand, referral patterns, audit management etc.). Otherwise, appropriate sounding terms may be chosen from at least three Read hierarchical trees making searches laborious (e.g. symptom codes beginning 16C.., an injury code beginning S57.., or a musculoskeletal code beginning N1. . .). The best approach is to use the terms 'backache', or 'low back pain' which will access symptom codes with the stem 16C. . . If a firm diagnosis is made at a later stage, this can be added (e.g acute disc prolapse, scoliosis) without compromising the ability to examine the prevalence of back pain and associated rate of sickness certification, referral patterns etc.

Box 4: Camden and Islington audit of GP practice before and after intervention

Camden and Islington MAAG sent 227 GPs a postal questionnaire in July 1997, held educational meetings and issued GPs with laminated copies of guidelines, then sent a repeat questionnaire in February 1998. Response rate was 60 per cent. Results are shown as percentage of GPs complying with recommendations before and after the educational meetings:

Not advising bed rest, 35%/51%;
Advising normal activity, 25%/34%;
Advising regular analgesia, 50%/54%;
Would request X-ray within 4 weeks of onset, 29%/23%;
Would refer for root pain of <4 weeks, 30%/13%;
Would refer for gait disturbance, 58%/61%;
Would refer for other red flags – all 90–99% at baseline, and small increase.

Patient-centred strategies

In the wider context, many studies of the provision of computerized patient information, treatment planners or interactive education show resultant improved care.[7] Manual reminder systems have been less studied.

The need for good patient information in back pain is illustrated by the results of a small audit of patient expectations conducted by Camden and Islington MAAG. Many patients with acute LBP entered the GP surgery expecting an X-ray (22 per cent) and specialist referral (20 per cent). Both these issues are specifically addressed by *The Back Book*, the self-help booklet produced by the RCGP to accompany the guidelines, and by an RCGP back pain poster.

The Back Book is also likely to be an effective tool for GPs wanting to give positive messages and clear advice about avoiding disability. Before being issued it was carefully piloted and found to be well received by patients, in contrast to many health professionals who feared that the books strong 'help yourself' message would seem unsympathetic.

Unfortunately at the time of writing only 110 000 copies had been purchased from the suppliers, which may reflect in part the relatively high cost of the product (60p per copy when bought in bulk). This cost has to be borne by GPs if they are to comply with the regulations of the 'Red Book' which determines what services and items patients can or cannot be charged for. In Oxfordshire, an alternative patient information leaflet (Northamptonshire GriPP back pain advice leaflet) was identified and reproduced at very low cost, and GPs were encouraged to use this, if reluctant to hand out copies of *The Back Book* (but see below in *Social Cognition Model*).

Mass media campaigns

Several studies demonstrate that mass media campaigns affect health services utilization. If political will were to ensure funding, and professionals in the field were in agreement, a mass media campaign might have a reasonable impact in the UK.

Resources

Adequate resources might seem an obvious accompaniment to any new national guidelines but are, in fact, commonly missing. The RCGP guidelines are no exception, and some implicit requirements like rapid access to physiotherapists with appropriate training in back care and manipulation, or affordable access to other manipulative therapists, are by no means universal throughout the various health authority regions or primary care groups.

To date, only one cost analysis of NHS provision of cross-disciplinary care has been identified.[4] Wiltshire Health Authority undertook a study of 344 patients compared with 194 matched historical controls. Application of the CSAG 1994 recommendations and provision of early manipulative therapy cost £126 per patient giving a total cost of £43 500 (encompassing a small increase in analgesia costs and a 25 per cent increase in X-rays as a result of chiropractic policy) but was associated with 20 per cent fewer GP consultations, an unquantified reduction in secondary care referrals, and a reduction in Med 5 certified days equivalent to a saving of £54 000. An important conclusion by the study's authors was that GPs follow guidelines if adequately resourced.

Understanding the psychology of implementation

An understanding of the determinants of whether and when a professional changes practice may be gained from behavioural science and some models used to describe behavioural change.

Stage model of behaviour

This is probably the best known model, sometimes known as the 'cycle of change' and frequently used in the context of influencing patients' smoking habit or other lifestyle choices. It can also be applied to health professionals asked to change their practice.[7] Thus individuals are thought to pass through a sequence of stages and the kinds of interventions needed at different stages vary.

In the first stage – *pre-contemplation* – no reason for change has been given. For instance a GP may believe that mechanical back pain is a condition over which he has little influence; that provided he recognizes pathology he is doing his job; and that if he offers a 'reassuring' X-ray or other imaging technique, some strong analgesics, recommends bed rest and gives a sick note he has served the patient's interests as best he can.

In this pre-contemplation phase, just some very basic information about the potential harm of this approach may be required to facilitate transition to the contemplation phase. Some practitioners may need to be shocked by, for instance, the view that,

> 'Prolonged disability from low back injury is aided and abetted by the health care provision system in general, and by doctors and physiotherapists in particular.'[10]

This view (which is far from proven!) should make practitioners want to examine their approach in the light of current evidence.

In the next stage – the *contemplation phase* – the clinician might be thinking through difficult areas, such as,

> 'How am I going to persuade a patient that the best course is to ignore the pain, keep active, mask pain if necessary with regular analgesics, and above all keep moving. Am I really going to tell a brick-layer with severe LBP that he should stay at work . . .?'.

Next comes the *preparation stage* – when the clinician might seek to satisfy himself that the recommendations are sound by accessing the evidence, or discussing with an expert the risks of prolonged bed-rest or sick certification.[11] He might access some evidence-based patient information leaflets to reinforce his verbal message to the patient, might find a poster or a text book photograph illustrating good and bad posture, bending and lifting techniques for manual labourers, and might speak to local physiotherapists about how to ensure patients are fit for their job of work.

The *action stage* – when the new approach is put into practice, will follow if the previous stage goes well.

For the new management approach to continue – *maintenance* – reminders may be required. Exposure to another set of gloomy statistics about time off with back pain might serve this purpose! Alternatively, a GP might see a patient who has joined his practice from elsewhere who tells him that he is crippled by 'degenerative disc disease' has a lumbar X-ray 'full of bony abnormalities' and who has taken his sick role so seriously he wears a plaster cast jacket, avoids activity and draws maximum disability benefits. This patient should remind the GP to avoid damning medical jargon, and be pro-active in patients who have psychosocial factors placing them at risk of chronicity.

Learning theory

This model emphasizes how probability of behaving in a certain way is positively or negatively reinforced by experience or environmental influences. If for instance, the first patient with recurrent LBP that you, a GP, refers to a chiropractor returns to you commenting positively about the short duration of this back pain episode and no loss of work, then positive reinforcement of that behaviour occurs. By contrast, if you try recommending to a patient that he takes paracetamol at regular six hourly intervals and he subsequently rings back to say the regime does not touch the pain, the experience will tend to erode (negatively reinforce) your new prescribing practice. It is worth noting that negative experiences early on in a new behaviour have a particularly powerful reinforcing effect.

Social cognition model

This model emphasizes that behaviour is shaped, not so much by environmental influences as by beliefs, attitudes and intentions.[6]

Perceived benefits are weighed against perceived barriers, commonly the benefit of improved outcome versus the cost of change. So for instance, before GPs dismiss *The Back Book* as too expensive, they should be encouraged to weigh up the following;

> 'If I identify a patient with biopsychosocial risk factors for chronic back pain, and I give or lend them a copy of The Back Book at my surgery's expense, might this help save me repeated consultations as well as the patient's misery?'

Whether someone changes their behaviour is also dependent on perceptions about the attitudes of important others. For instance, a GP may question,

> 'Will I be viewed negligent if I refer a patient with a spinal tumour or a vertebral fracture to an osteopath?'

These 'important others' may include GP colleagues, secondary care services, medical defence organisations, or the manipulative therapist in question. For many GPs or consultants to start referring patients to osteopaths and chiropractors requires understanding of the professional and legal liability issues (see Boxes 5 and 6).

Box 5: Legal liability

'In the event of a mishap directly resulting from an alternative practitioner's intervention, UK medical defence bodies would, in general, resist any attempt to attribute liability to a GP. However, if the GP had referred the patient to a practitioner with a poor track record, then the GP might be deemed reckless, and liability might be shared.'

Medical Defence Union, 1996

Box 6: Professional liability (good medical practice, duties of a doctor, GMC 1998)

Para 39. Delegation involves asking a nurse, doctor, medical student or other healthcare worker to provide treatment or care on your behalf. When you delegate care or treatment you must be sure that the person to whom you delegate is competent to undertake the procedure or therapy involved. You will still be responsible for the overall management of the patient.

Para 40. Referral involves transferring some or all of the responsibility for the patient's care, usually temporarily and for a particular purpose, such as additional investigation, care or treatment, which falls outside your competence. Usually you will refer patients to another registered medical practitioner. If this is not the case, you must be satisfied that such healthcare workers are accountable to a statutory regulatory body, and that a registered medical practitioner, usually a general practitioner, retains overall responsibility for the patient.

Also important is 'self-efficacy' – the belief in one's ability to perform a particular behaviour;

> *'I will recommend staying active, avoiding bed rest and once the patient is recovering, taking general conditioning exercise, because I believe I have adequately excluded significant pathology.'*

Attitudes to guidelines

For professionals to embrace guidelines enthusiastically requires an understanding of their role in day-to-day patient care. Evidence-based medicine is not 'cook-book' medicine, and guidelines need to be applied sensitively to individual patients.

'Good doctors use both clinical expertise and the best available external evidence, and neither alone is enough. Without an individual's clinical expertise, practice risks becoming evidence-tyrannized, for even excellent external evidence may be inapplicable or inappropriate for individual patients. Without best available evidence, practice risks becoming rapidly out of date to the detriment of patient-care.'
Centre for Evidence-Based Medicine, Oxford

References

1. Waddell, G., Feder, G., McIntosh, A. *et al.* (1996). *Clinical Guidelines for the Management of Acute Low Back Pain*. London. Royal College of General Practitioners.
2. Roland, M., Waddell, G., Klaber, XXX., Moffett, J. *et al.* (1997). *The Back Book*. The Stationery Office, London.
3. Cluzeau, F., Littlejohns, P., Grimshaw, J., Feder, G. (1999). Development and application of a generic methodology to assess the quality of clinical guidelines. *Int. J. Qual. Health Care*, **11**(1), 21–28.
4. Hibble, A., Kanka, D., Pencheon, D., Pooles, F. (1998). Guidelines in general practice: the new Tower of Babel? *BMJ*, **317**, 862–863.
5. Scheurmier, N., Breen, A. (1998). A pilot study of the purchase of manipulation services for acute back pain in the United Kingdom. *J. Manip. Physiol. Ther.*, **21**(1), 14–18.
6. http://www.doh.gov.uk.public/backpain/htm.
7. Effective Health Care. Getting Evidence into Practice (1999). NHS Centre for Reviews and Dissemination, University of York, York. The Royal Society of Medicine Press Ltd.
9. Grol, R. (1997). Personal paper. Beliefs and evidence in clinical practice.*BMJ*, **315**, 418–421.
10. Spitzer, W.O. (1993). Low back pain in the workplace: Attainable benefits not attained. *Br. J. Ind. Med.*, **50**(5), 385–388.

Glossary

Aerobic re-conditioning
Training programme designed to improve cardiovascular fitness and physical strength.

Annulus fibrosis
Concentric layers of fibrous tissue surrounding the nucleus pulposus of the intervertebral disc.

Arnold-Chiari malformation
Congenital disorder in which there is distortion of the base of the skull with protrusion of the lower brainstem and parts of the cerebellum through the opening for the spinal cord at the base of the skull. Often associated with neural tube defects and hydrocephalus.

Axial (view)
Looking along the axis of the body or spine. In MRI this is a 'worm's eye' view i.e. looking from underneath upwards.

Brachialgia
Nerve root pain in upper limb.

Cauda equina
Lower part of spinal cord composed of long strands or filaments commencing at about L1/L2.

Chemonucleolysis
Injection of chymopapain to reduce disc herniation.

Cobb angle
The angle between the upper border of the upper end vertebra and the lower border of the lower end vertebra. In practice this means 0° is straight. Thirty degrees is noticeable, 50° is bad enough for an operation and 90° or more is severe.

Cognitive (behavioural) therapy
A form of psychotherapy based on the interpretation of situations that determine how an individual feels and behaves. Based on the premise that cognition, the process of acquiring knowledge and forming beliefs, is a primary determinant of mood and behaviour. It aims to correct negative thinking which is at the root of aberrant behaviour.

Coronal (view)
Through body from front to back.

CT/CAT scan computerized (axial) tomography
Radiographic technique that uses a computer to assimilate multiple X-ray images into a two-dimensional cross-sectional image. Dye may be injected to enhance clarification.

Decompression (spinal)
Reducing the pressure on a nerve root by enlarging the area or space around it. Discectomy is a form on its own, but in spinal stenosis bone and soft tissues including the ligamentum flavum are also removed.

Dermatome
The area of skin supplied by a single spinal nerve.

Diastematomyelia
A bony or fibrous spur dividing the vertebral canal in the sagittal plane.

Discectomy
Partial (usually) or complete removal of an intervertebral disc.

Discitis
Infection or inflammation of an intervertebral disc or disc space.

Discogenic (pain)
Pain originating from a disc.

Discography
Injection of contrast into an intervertebral disc in order to provoke familiar discogenic pain in patients being considered for spinal fusion and thus to confirm or refute the source of back pain.

Dorsal root ganglion
Area where posterior (dorsal) and anterior (ventral) branches merge to form peripheral nerve.

Enthesitis
Inflammation resulting from stress on muscle or tendon attached to bone.

Facet joint
One of a pair of hinged joints between vertebra.

Filum terminali
Slender tapering terminal section of the spinal cord.

FRP/functional restoration programme
Progressive exercise rehabilitative regimen often used in conjunction with cognitive behavioural therapy in the management of chronic low back pain.

Haemangioma
Congenital anomaly in which there is a proliferation of blood vessels which may form a tumour-like mass.

Instrumentation
Insertion of metalwork; plates, screws, pins, etc. e.g. in a spinal fusion.

Joint (usually facet) block
Injection of anaesthetic to 'block out' pain from joint and which may be used to confirm source of back pain.

Kyphoscoliosis
Kyphosis and scoliosis occurring together.

Kyphosis
Excessive curvature of the spine in the sagittal plane.

Laminectomy
Removal of lamina enabling access to disc at operation.

Laminotomy
Removal of only part of the lamina to gain access to disc.

Lateral recess stenosis
A decrease in size of the lateral recess – the area bounded by the pedicle, the superior articular facet, the posterior lateral surface of the vertebral body and the intervertebral disc. Bony hypertrophy of the superior facet, postero-lateral osteophytes, or a far lateral disc herniation can cause nerve root entrapment.

Lateral stenosis
Nerve root compression as it exits the neural foramen. The nerve root is compressed because of the superior articular facet or migration of the facet upward.

Lhermitte's sign
Pain and tingling (electric shocks) in extremes of flexion and extension of the neck where the diameter of the cervical spinal cord is reduced as a result of for example a spinal tumour.

Lordosis
Excessive curvature of the spine in the sagittal plane (apex anteriorly).

Lower motor neuron/lesion
Nerve arising from the anterior horn cell of the spinal cord where it joins with (synapse) the upper motor neuron of the corticospinal tract. From the anterior horn cell it leaves the cord as the anterior nerve root then enters a peripheral nerve supplying motor function to a group of muscles called a myotome.

Meta-analysis
A statistical technique which summarizes the results of several studies into a single estimate, giving more weight to results from larger studies.

Myelogram
Radiography of spinal cord after injection of radio-opaque substance into the spinal arachnoid space.

Myelopathy
Compression of the spinal cord or cauda equina.

Pars defect
A lesion or fracture of the pars interaricularis.

Pars interarticularis
Part of the posterior elements of the vertebral body forming part of the neural arch.

Radicular
Along a single nerve root e.g. pain.

Radiculopathy
Compression of a single nerve root.

RCT/randomized controlled trial
A research trial in which subjects are randomly assigned to two groups: one (the experimental group) receiving the intervention – treatment, operation etc., to be tested – and the other (comparison or controls) receiving an alternative treatment or none at all. The two groups are then compared to assess the effectiveness of the intervention.

Sagittal
Anterior-posterior view.

Spinal stenosis
Narrowing of the spinal canal.

Scheurmann's disease (adolescent kyphosis)
Osteochondritis of the epiphyseal vertebra end plates in children usually at puberty often causing kyphosis backache and characteristic disc herniations or Schmorl's nodes.

Scoliosis
Curvature of the spine in the coronal plane.

Sensitivity
Measure of a high proportion of true cases. A high level is desirable and indicates that the test is not missing cases.

Specificity
Measure of how reliable a test is in only being positive when it should be. A high level is desirable and means that there are very few false positives.

Spondyloarthritis
Arthritis of the spine.

Spondylolisthesis
A forward slip of a vertebra relative to the vertebra below.

Spondylolysis
Defect in pars interarticularis of a vertebra.

Structural curve
A curve of the spine which cannot be corrected in a supine bending film.

TENS – transcutaneous nerve stimulation
A physical method for relieving pain using electrical impulses to the skin.

Upper motor neuron/lesion
Nerve that runs from the motor cortex of the brain along the corticospinal (pyramidal) tracts crossing to the other side of the cord as it does to join with (synapse) the anterior horn cells of the spinal cord. Damage can occur to it anywhere between the cortex and anterior horn cell.

Abbreviations

AHCPR, Agency for Health Care Policy and Research
AS, ankylosing spondylitis
BMD, bone mineral density
CNS, central nervous system
CSAG, Clinical Standards Advisory Group
CSF, cerebrospinal fluid
CT, computerized tomography
CVA, cerebrovascular accident
DSS, Department of Social Security
ESR, erythrocyte sedimentation rate
FBC, full blood count
FRP, functional restoration programme
GA, general anaesthetic
GP, general practitioner
IV, intravenous
LA, local anaesthetic
LBP, lower back pain
LD, lumbar decompression
LMN, lower motor neuron
MRC, Medical Research Council
MRI, magnetic resonance imaging
NSAID, non-steroidal anti-inflammatory drug
OI, osteogenesis imperfecta
PCG, primary care groups
PCR, polymerase chain reaction
PCT, primary care trusts
PSA, prostatic specific antigen
PsA, psoriatic arthritis
ReA, reactive arthritis
SLR, slight leg raise
SSRI, serotonin re-uptake inhibitor
TCA, tricyclic antidepressants
UMN, upper motor neuron
VHL, von Hippel-Lindau disease

Index

Abdominal syndrome, 100
Achondroplasia, 105, 110
Acupuncture, 167
Aerobic re-conditioning, 189
Alkaptonuria, 105, 111
Anal tone and sensation, 66
Ankylosing spondylitis, 6, 81, 82, 84, 140
    Bath index, 84
    drug treatment, 86–7
    exercises, 86
    family history, 83
    history, 83
    HLA-B27 status, 85, 140
Annulus fibrosis, 189
Antidepressants, 51, 149
Aortic aneurysm, 142
Arnold–Chiari malformation, 189
Astrocytoma, 91, 97
Audit, 182–3
Axial view, 189

'Back Book', 41, 184
Back pain syndrome, 100
Back Schools, 166, 168
Bath Ankylosing Spondylitis Index, 84
Behavioural change, 185–7
Biofeedback, 167
Bone density charts, 106
Bone donor pain, 159–60
Bowel function, 66
Bowstring test, 59, 60
Brachialgia, 189
Bracing, 116
Brown–Sequard syndrome, 94–5
Brucellosis, 103

Calcitonin, 76, 157
Cauda equina syndrome, 64–6, 189
    bowel function, 66
    characteristics, 8, 64–5
    incidence, 66
    lower limb dysfunction, 66
    management, 66

saddle anaesthesia, 66
    urinary symptoms, 65
Cavernoma, 92, 97
Cervical syndromes, 94
Chemonucleolysis, 62, 64, 135, 157, 189
Chiropractic, 163–4
Chondrodysplasias, 105, 110
Chronic low back pain:
    drug therapy, 151
    premorbid factors, 15
    referral, 17–18, 24
    rehabilitation, 46–52
Cobb angle, 112, 189
Cognitive behavioural therapy, 48, 50, 189
Colchicine, 150
Compression paraplegia, 89
Computed tomography (CT), 95, 129–30,
    156, 189
Consultation patterns, 22–3
Continuing professional education, 180–1
Conus, 94
Coronal view, 189
Corticosteroids, 150
COX 2 inhibitors, 148
Cutaneous nerve damage, 161

Decompression, 158, 190
Deformity, see Spinal deformity
Dermatomes, 61, 190
Dermoids, 92
Diastematomyelia, 190
Diclofenac, 87
Disability, 20–2, 35–6
Disc prolapse, 154–5, 157
Disc space infection, 101–2
Discectomy, 157–8, 190
Discitis, 141, 190
Discogenic pain, 190
Discography, 135, 156, 190
Dorsal root ganglion, 190
Drug therapy, 50–1, 86–7, 147–52
Duchenne muscular dystrophy, 118
Duodenal ulcer, 142

Enthesitis, 190
Ependymoma, 91, 96, 97
Epidermoids, 92
Epidural abscess, 102–3, 141
Epidural steroids, 157
Evidence-based practice, 35
Exercises, 46, 47–9, 86, 166–7
  compliance, 48, 49

Facet joint, 190
  blocks, 134, 190
  pain, 132–3, 134
    neurotomy for, 135–6
Feedback, 182–3
Femoral stretch test, 60
Fibrous dysplasia, 109, 110–11
Filum terminali, 190
Forward bending test, 113, 114
Functional restoration programmes (FRPs),
  40, 47–50, 190
  efficacy, 49–50

Gout, 140
Guillain–Barré syndrome, 141
Gynaecological disorders, 142

Haemangioblastoma, 92, 97
Haemangioma, 190
Hip joint syndrome, 100
HLA-B27 status, 85, 140
Hyperparathyroidism, 105, 109, 110, 141

Iliac vessel aneurysm, 142
Incidence, 19
Infection, 6, 99–104, 140–1, 155
  differential diagnosis, 103
  postoperative, 160
Inflammatory diseases, 81–8
  examination, 83–4
  history, 82–3
  investigation, 84–5, 140
  management, 85–7
  prevalence, 81
Instrumentation, 190

Kyphoscoliosis, 191
Kyphosis, 121, 122, 191

Laboratory tests, 38, 139–43
Laminectomy, 191
Laminotomy, 191
Learning theory, 186
Lectures, 180–1
Leg pain, 'red flags', 58, 64
Legal liability, 187

Leukaemia, 141
Lhermitte's sign, 93, 94, 191
Local anaesthetic blocks, 134–5, 150
Lordosis, 191
Low back pain, *see* Chronic low back pain;
  Simple back pain
Lower motor neuron, 191
Lumbar disc herniation types, 63
Lumbar syndromes, 94

Magnetic resonance imaging (MRI), 95,
  130–7, 155–6
  contraindications, 131
  limited, 136–7
  therapeutic use, 134–6
Manipulation, 165–6
Marfan's syndrome, 105, 110
McCune Albright syndrome, 111
Mechanical back pain, 31, 155
Media campaigns, 184
Meningeal syndrome, 100
Meningioma, 91
Meta-analysis, 191
Metabolic disorders, 105–11, 141–2
Metalwork failure, 161
Metastatic disease, 90, 95, 96, 109, 141
Methyl methacrylate cement, 136
Motor power, 60–1, 62
MRC scale, 62
Multiple myeloma, 141
Muscle relaxants, 51, 148–9
Myelography, 156, 191
Myelopathy, 191

Neoplasia, 89–98, 155
  biopsy, 96
  classification, 89–90
  extradural, 90–1, 97
  extramedullary, 91, 97
  intramedullary, 91–2, 97
  investigation, 95, 141
  metastatic, 90, 95, 96, 109, 141
  prognosis, 97
  signs, 93–5
  symptoms, 92–3
  treatment, 96–7
Nerve root blocks, 134–5
Nerve root pain, 55–64, 156
  aetiology, 57–8
  investigation, 58–62
  leg pain, 58
  management, 10, 62, 64
  presentation, 55–7
  recurrence, 64
  and scoliosis, 56
  triaging, 7–9
Nerve root signs, 7
Neurofibromata, 91
Neurofibromatosis Type 1, 120

Neurogenic claudication, 9, 56, 68, 69–70
Night pain, 38, 58, 94
Non-steroidal anti-inflammatory drugs
(NSAIDs), 50, 86–7, 148
Non-union, 161

Opinion leaders, 182
Opioids, 149–50
Osteitis fribroa cystica, 110
Osteogenesis imperfecta, 105, 110
Osteomalacia, 105, 109–10
Osteomyelitis, 99–100, 140
Osteopathy, 163–4
Osteoporosis, 105, 107–8
Osteosclerosis, 109
Out-reach visits, 182

Paget's disease, 105, 108–9
Pain cycle, 46–7
Pain management, 40, 47
Pain Society of Great Britain and Northern
Ireland, 50
Pancreatitis, 142
Paracetamol, 147
Parathyroid bone disease, 105, 109, 110,
141
Pars defect, 133, 191
Patient information, 41, 184
Pedicle screws, 160
Percutaneous therapy, 135–6
Phenylbutasone, 148
Physical therapy, 163–70
referral for, 168
Physiotherapy, 40–1, 163, 164
specialist, 171–4
Porphyria, 142
Positive cross-over sign, 60
Postoperative complications, 159–61
Pott's disease, 102
Prevalence, 19–20
Prostatitis, 142
Psychosocial factors, 14–17, 32–4
'yellow flags', 3
Pyelonephritis, 142

Radicular/radiculopathy, 192
Radiology, 127–38
Randomized controlled trial, 192
Read codes, 183
'Red flags', 58, 75, 94, 103–4
Referred pain, 31, 38, 56
Reflexes, 60
Reiter's syndrome, 140
Reminder systems, 182
Resources, 184–5
Return to work, 16–17
Rhizolysis, 134

Root blocks, 134–5
Royal College of General Practitioners
(RCGP) guidelines, ix–x, 177–88
attitudes to, 187–8
dissemination, 179
implementation, 179–83, 185–7
success of, 178–80

Sacroiliac joint assessment, 84
Sacroiliitis, 81, 84
Saddle anaesthesia, 66
Sagittal view, 192
Salpingitis, 142
Scheurmann's disease, 121, 192
Schober's test, modified, 83–4
Scoliosis, 192
adolescent idiopathic, 112, 113, 114–17
benign neglect, 115
bracing, 116
exercises, 115
surgery, 117
congenital, 119–20
de novo (degenerative), 122
and nerve root pain, 56
neuromuscular (paralytic), 118
syndromal, 120
Selective serotonin re-uptake inhibitors
(SSRIs), 149
Sensory function, 60, 93–4
Simple back pain, xiv, 10–11, 29–45
and age, 30–1
consultation patterns, 22–3
and disability, 20–2, 35–6
economic costs of, 19
explaining to patients, 12–13
increase in cases of, 34–5
management, 11–12, 14, 39–44
timetable, 41–3, 168
mechanical, 31, 155
pathology, 29–30
premorbid factors, 15
prevalence, 19–20
prognosis, 32
referral, 13–14, 17
site of, 31
triage, 10–11, 36–9
Smoking, 34
Social cognition, 186–7
Spinal cord:
blood supply, 90
compression, 89, 93, 94–5
Spinal decompression, 158, 190
Spinal deformity, 112–23
in adults, 122
curve progression, 112
diagnosis, 114
examination, 113, 114
investigation, 114
terminology, 112
Spinal fusion, 158–9

Spinal neoplasia, *see* Neoplasia
Spinal stabilization, 158–9
Spinal stenosis, 68–77, 155, 192
  causes, 71
  central, 69
  classification, 71
  defined, 68–9
  differential diagnosis, 74–5
  epidemiology, 71–2
  investigation, 73–4
  lateral, 69,191
  lateral recess, 191
  mechanism, 70
  mixed, 69
  referral, 77
  signs, 72–3
  symptoms, 69–70, 72
  tandem, 69
  treatment, 75–6, 157
Spondyloarthropathies, 81, 140, 192, *see
  also* Inflammatory diseases
Spondylolisthesis, 6, 133, 192
Spondylolysis, 133, 192
Stage model, 185–6
Straight leg raise, 8, 58–60
Structural curve, 192
Sulphasalazine, 87
Surgery, 153–62
  complications, 159–61
  indications, 154, 156
  patient selection, 153
  prognosis, 153
Synovial cysts, 133

TENS, 167, 192
Test sensitivity/specificity, 192
Thoracic syndromes, 94
Traction, 168
Triage, 5–9, 10–11, 14–17, 36–9
Tricyclic antidepressants, 51, 149
Trigger point injections, 150
Tuberculosis, 102
Tumours, *see* Neoplasia

'Up going' plantar responses, 93
Upper motor neuron, 93, 192
Urinary symptoms, 8, 65

Vascular claudication, 9
Vertebral collapse:
  investigation, 133
  methyl methacrylate cement, 136
Vertebral osteomyelitis, 99–100, 140
Vitamin D, 109
Von Hipple Lindau disease, 92
Von Recklinghausen's syndrome, 120

Waddell signs, 33, 154

X-rays (plain), 38, 128–9, 156

'Yellow flags', 3